Polarized:

Carl Jung,
Jordan Peterson,
Samuel Hahnemann,
Greta Thunberg, and
the Devouring Mother
are going to a party

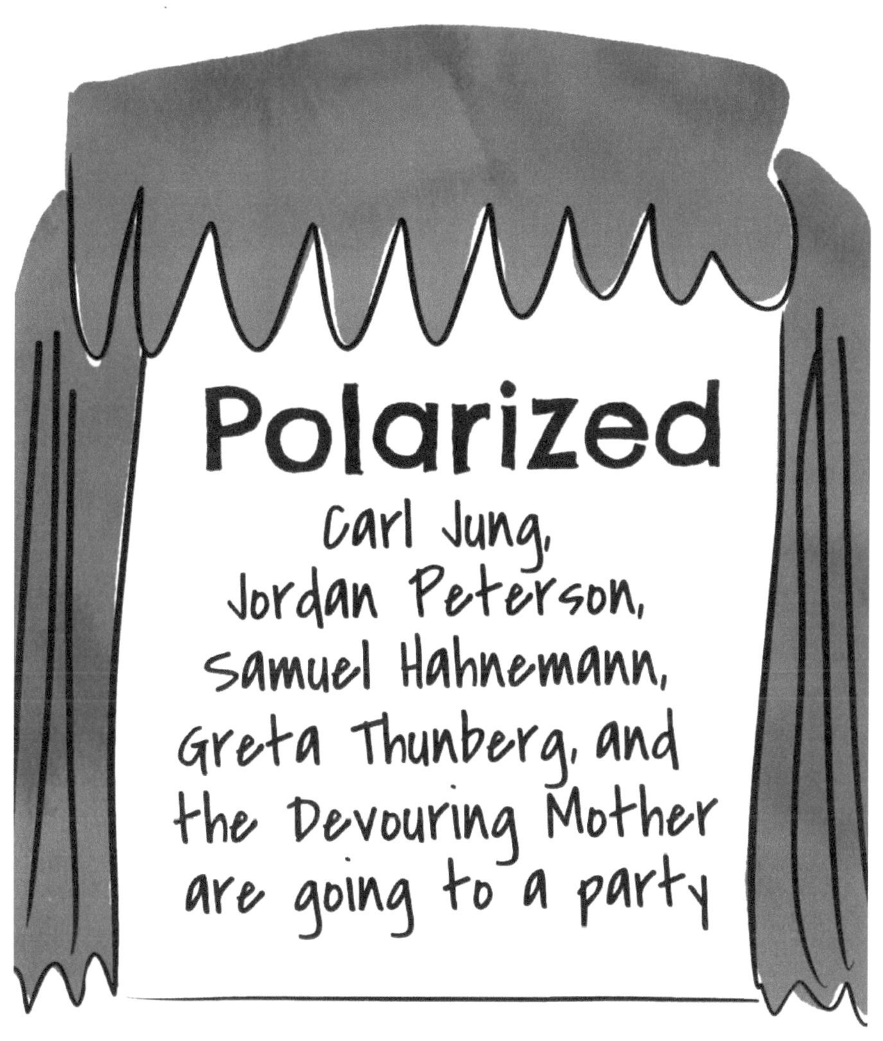

By Misna Burelli and Lena Kratz

Library of Congress Cataloging-in-Publication Data available on file.

ISBN 978-1-7342928-0-0

Cover design by ImmuneAdvantage, LLC

Thinking is difficult

.

That is why most people judge

.

Carl Jung

Dedicated to all people who think

.

Acknowledgments

Thank you
to all of you who
contributed to this project
.

Table of Contents

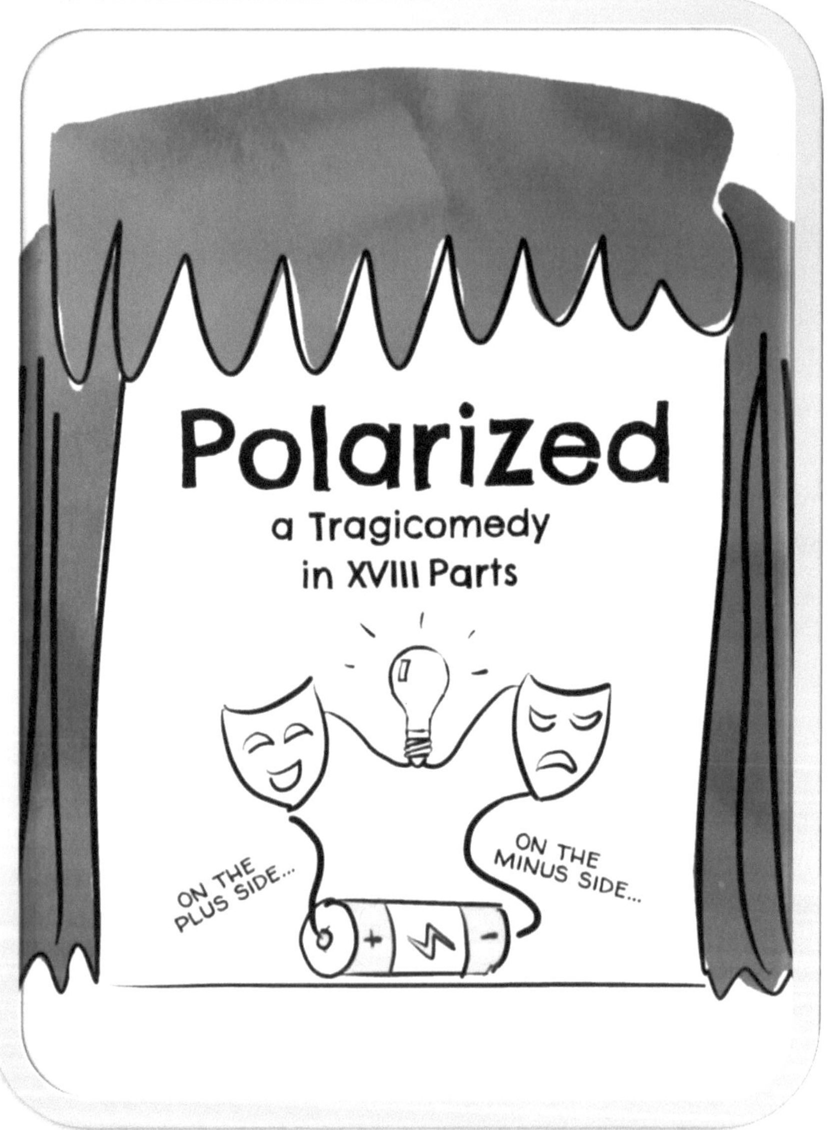
Polarized
a Tragicomedy
in XVIII Parts
ON THE
PLUS SIDE...
ON THE
MINUS SIDE...
+
-

Introduction

By Misna Burelli

Everything is connected. But the dots are often far apart, and much of the time it feels like traveling through a maze to go from A to B. It is like being back at my birthday party as a child, playing the game of telephone. The game begins with whispering a secret word into one child's ear. The child is supposed to transfer the message to the next child, and so on until it reaches the last person who reveals it. Most of the time the word is so scrambled by the transfer process that a new word is produced, which has nothing in common with the original word. It is a pretty funny game.

But sometimes I feel that this is exactly what has been happening in our world. Information doesn't flow smoothly—it gets stuck. News of great discoveries only get spread within small research circles and don't reach other fields. From the flow of information to personal relationships or scientific discoveries, it's often difficult to connect dots that should be connected. But once it happens, it feels completely natural.

So how can we facilitate the process? That's a really big question! What follows is an attempt to do just that, by encouraging a discussion between people who should have met—everyone is invited to contribute parts to the complicated puzzle!

Let's have a party, but at *this* party, let's put all cards on the table! If you have something to contribute, we would love to hear from you. Send your Tweets to @LenaandMisna. We are looking forward to some interesting discussions!

Cast of Characters

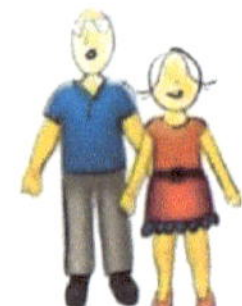

MISNA BURELLI AND LENA KRATZ

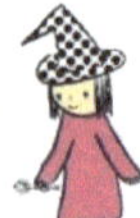

THE DEVOURING MOTHER

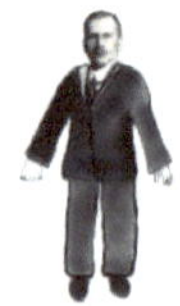

DR. CARL JUNG

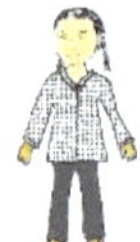

GRETA THUNBERG

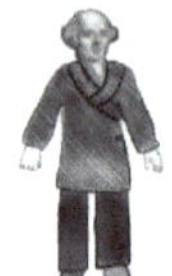

DR. SAMUEL HAHNEMANN

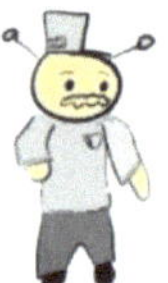

GENERAL FAIRFITE

COMMANDER OF THE IMMUNE SYSTEM ARMY

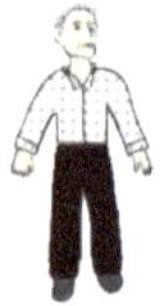

DR. JORDAN PETERSON

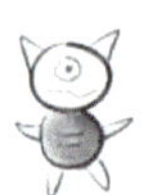

AL EHRGY IMMUNE SYSTEM TEACHING ASSISTANT

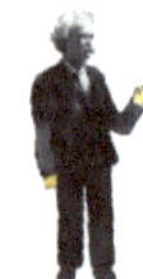

MARK TWAIN

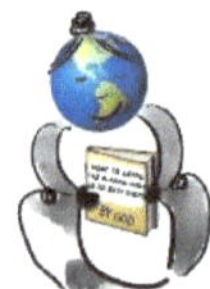

MOTHER NATURE

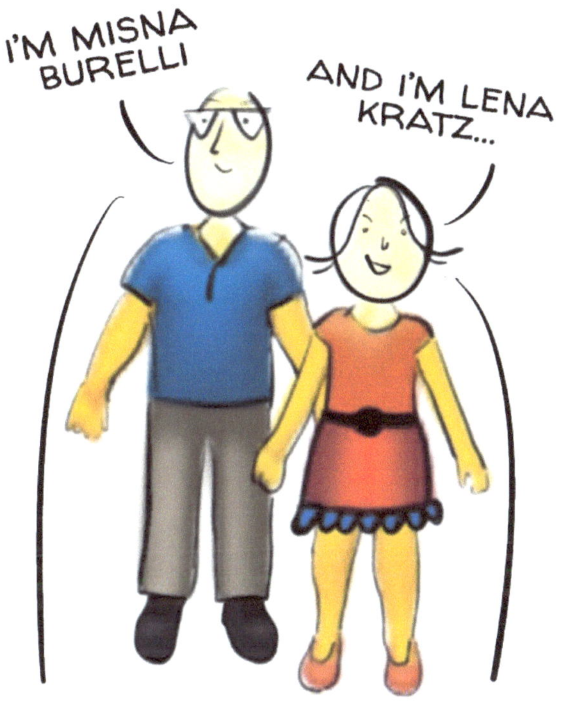

AND WE ARE YOUR HOSTS THIS EVENING...

ENJOY THE SHOW!

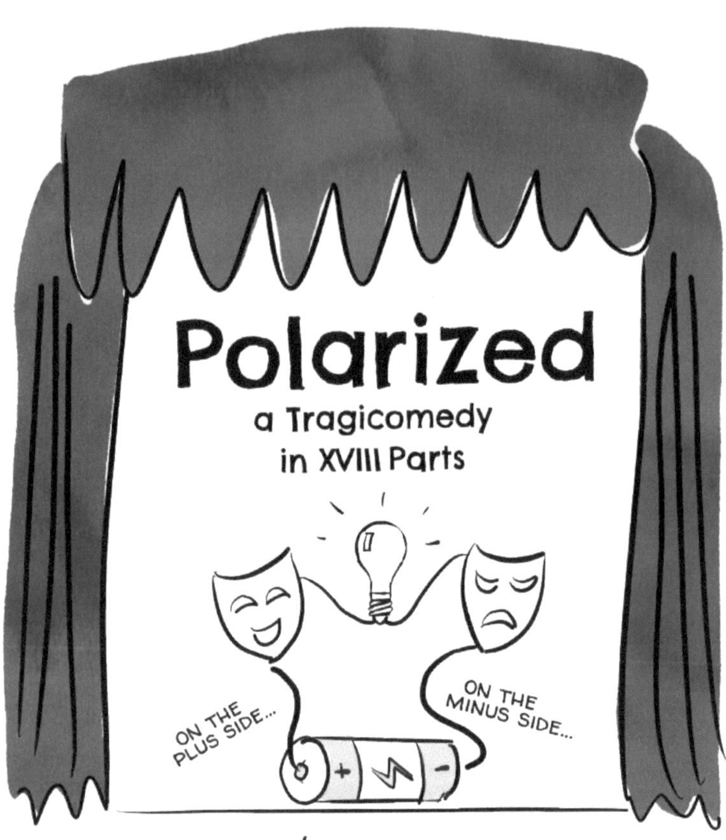
Polarized
a Tragicomedy
in XVIII Parts
ON THE PLUS SIDE...
ON THE MINUS SIDE...

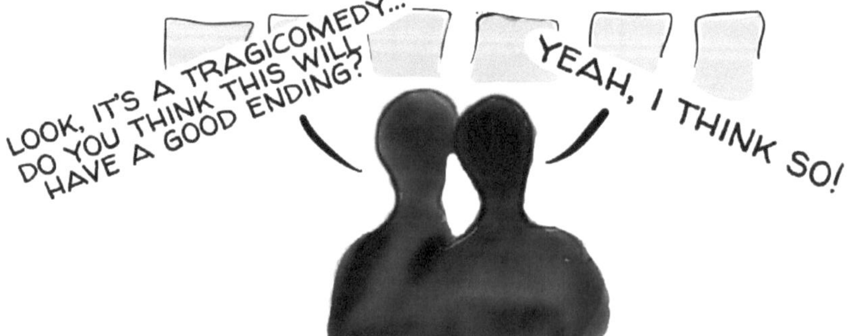
LOOK, IT'S A TRAGICOMEDY... DO YOU THINK THIS WILL HAVE A GOOD ENDING?
YEAH, I THINK SO!

…it all began one beautiful summer
evening…

with Mother Nature sitting
in her library…

…thinking about the future…

WE SHOULD HAVE A PARTY…
LENA AND MISNA CAN ORGANIZE IT…
WE NEED SOME GOOD DISCUSSIONS
AND SOME BRAINSTORMING…
HOW TO LEVEL THE PLAYING FIELD IN 10 EASY STEPS
BY GOD
Thinking Outside The Box
When Your Human is Not Listening

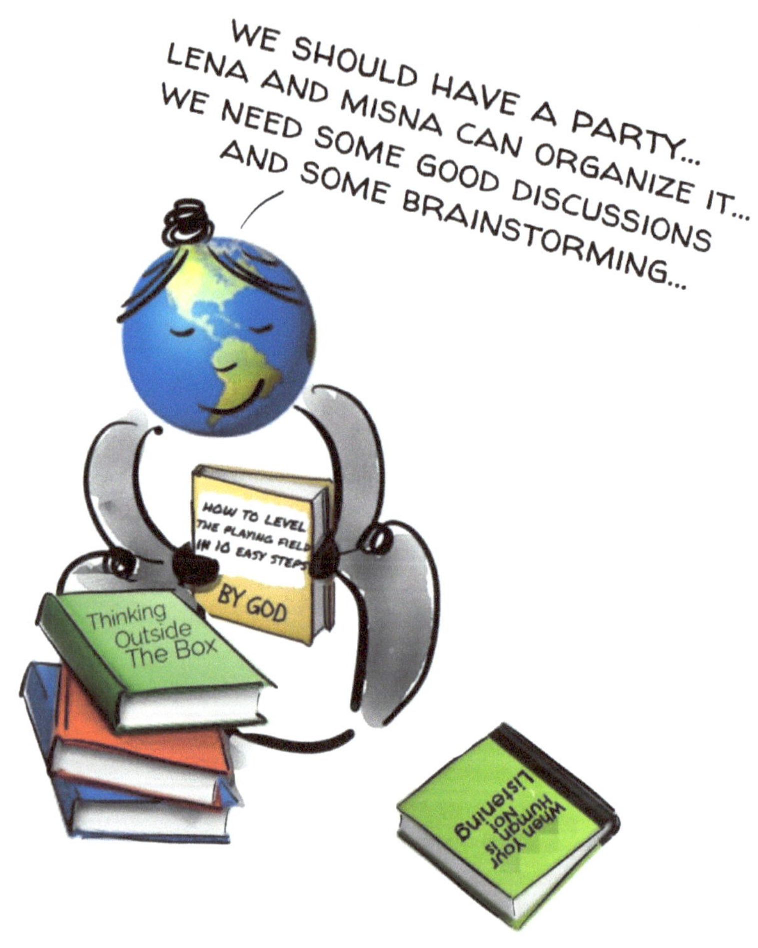

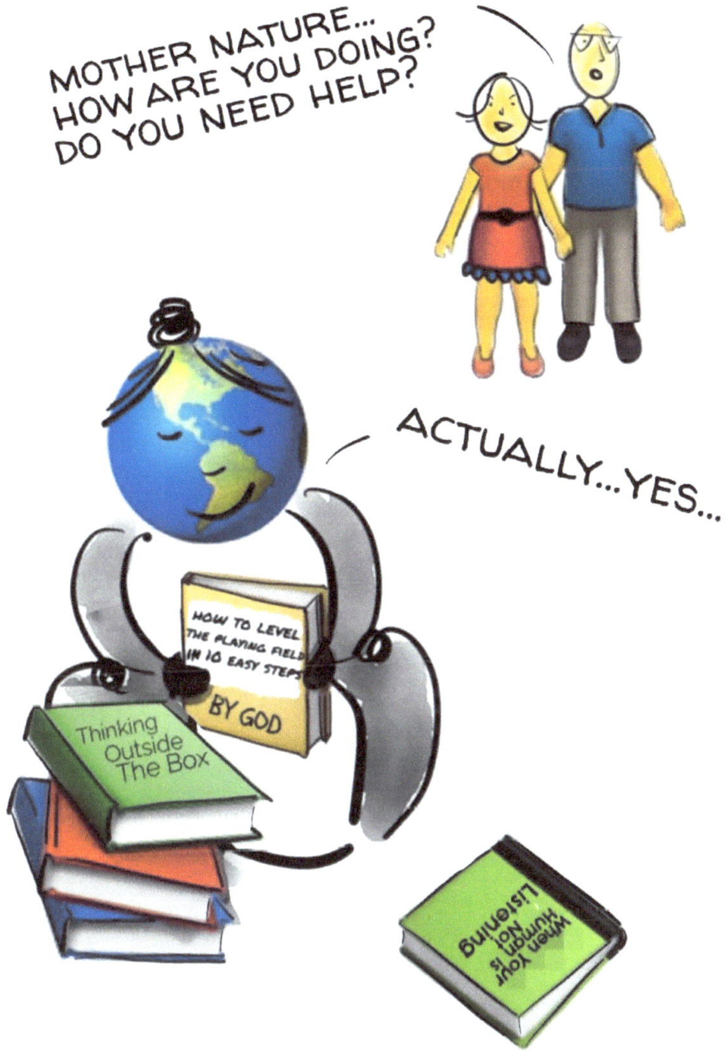
MOTHER NATURE...
HOW ARE YOU DOING?
DO YOU NEED HELP?
ACTUALLY...YES...
HOW TO LEVEL THE PLAYING FIELD IN 10 EASY STEPS
BY GOD
Thinking Outside The Box
When Your Human is Not Listening

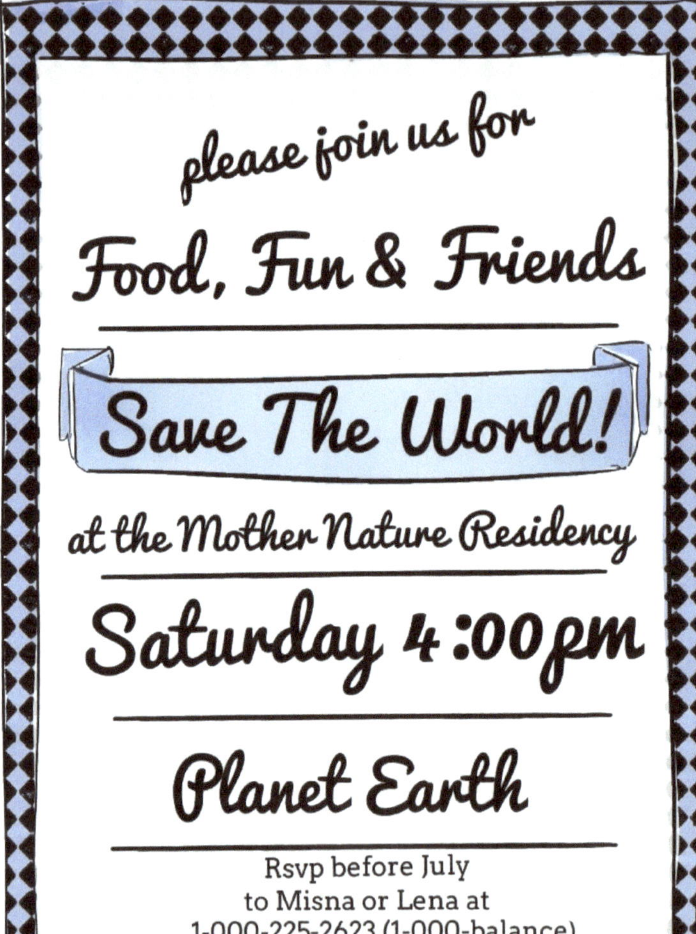
please join us for
Food, Fun & Friends
Save The World!
at the Mother Nature Residency
Saturday 4:00pm
Planet Earth
Rsvp before July
to Misna or Lena at
1-000-225-2623 (1-000-balance)

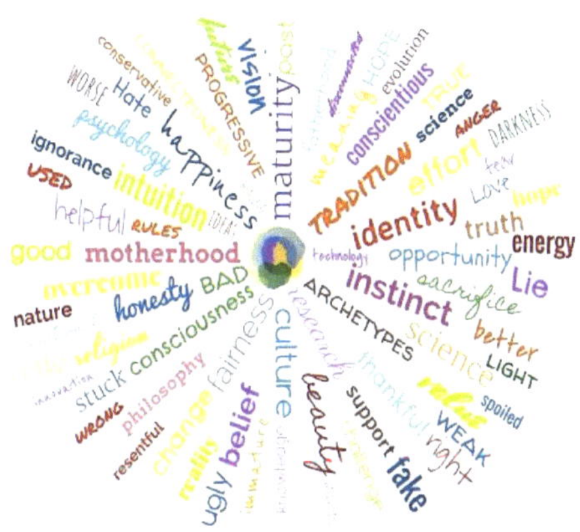
maturity
vision
PROGRESSIVE
conservative
WORSE
Hate
psychology
happiness
ignorance
USED
intuition
helpful
RULES
good
motherhood
honesty
BAD
nature
consciousness
stuck
philosophy
WRONG
resentful
change
fairness
ugly
belief
culture
research
beauty
support
fake
thankful
right
WEAK
spoiled
LIGHT
science
ARCHETYPES
better
instinct
sacrifice
Lie
opportunity
energy
truth
identity
technology
TRADITION
effort
Love
hope
DARKNESS
ANGER
science
TRUE
conscientious
evolution
HOPE

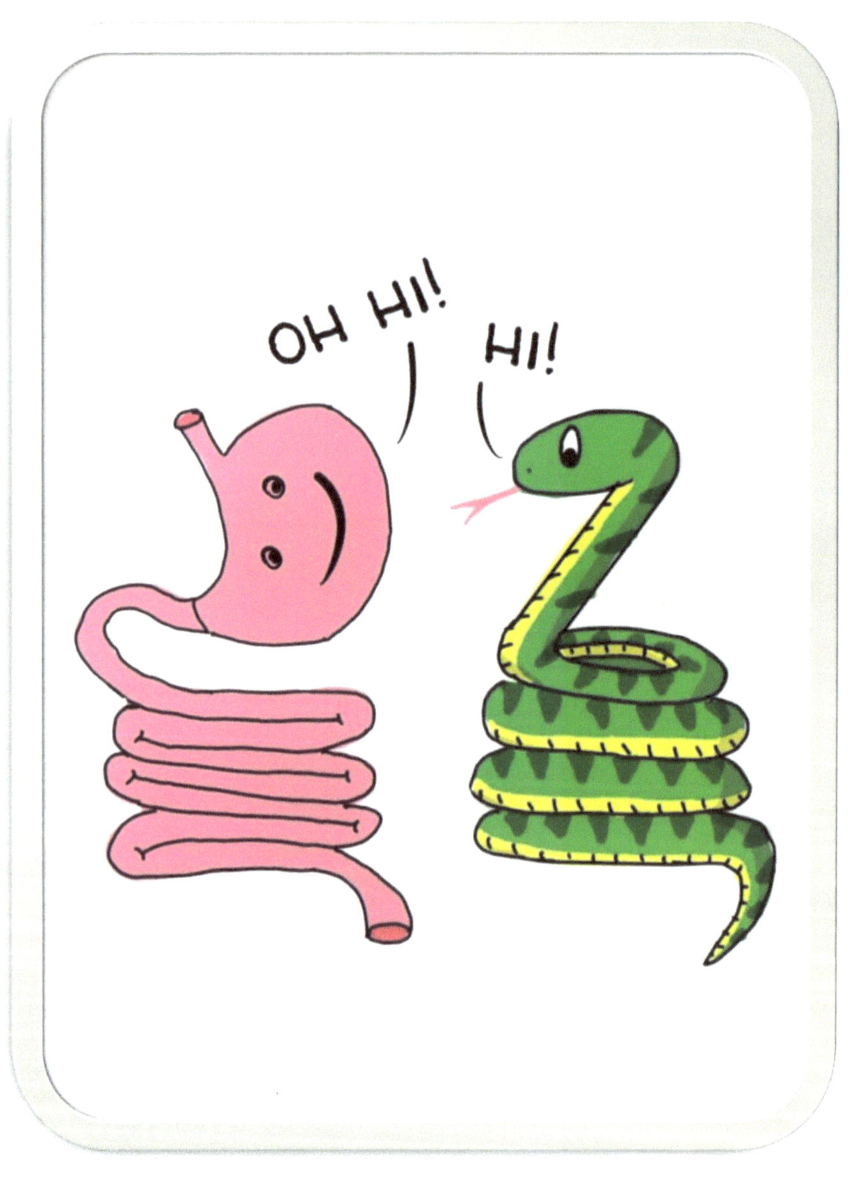
OH HI!
HI!

Diet and Health

By Lena Kratz

When my husband Misna and I graduated with doctorate degrees in analytical chemistry back in the '90s, we had no idea what was to come. We were looking forward to a life without studying and staying up late—no more researching difficult concepts! I joined a pharmaceutical company and started my career there. Misna did the same. It all seemed straightforward and easy!

The time I started thinking for real came when Jackie, one of our two children, did not develop proper language skills at the age of two. Her pediatrician completely brushed it off, deeming it as well within the normal range. Jackie had been a finicky child for a while—suffering from a stomach condition known as reflux, which required extensive medical testing, including a nasal endoscopy. This unpleasant procedure involved steering a camera down her nose and throat. The resulting pictures gave the all-clear, but we, as parents, were upset and worried. I had suffered from heartburn for years, and, knowing how painful it could be, felt miserable for her. But there was something else that troubled me even more: *how could a baby suffer from reflux?* I had never heard of such a thing!

The doctor said not to worry, stating that this was quite common. Most kids outgrew their symptoms by kindergarten. We were surprised to learn that this condition was widespread—*it didn't make sense*—stirring up discomfort in me. It was even more puzzling to hear about children taking acid blockers for reflux. How could this be common in small children?

But now we had an even bigger problem. Even though the doctor denied my suspicions, I could sense that Jackie was speech delayed. Were the poor language skills and the reflux condition *related?*

Shortly after, our older daughter Emily suddenly began sleepwalking. At eleven years old, she was far older than a typical child suffering from night terrors. The problem was accompanied by a range of unexpected symptoms: sudden milk intolerance, rapid tooth decay—

one tooth deteriorated so badly that it had to be pulled—and an allergy to pistachios. *What was going on?*

Again, the doctor brushed it all off as "no big deal", "many kids have these issues" and even "I also had that in college and people thought it was hilarious". *Really?!* According to him, our best option to deal with the issue was prescription medication. We knew all about this kind of treatment, and it didn't sound great. In fact, one of our friends, suffering from the same ailment, always took a pill before going to bed because he had once woken up from a sleepwalking episode hanging over a balcony. *Scary!*

Overnight, our whole family became a complete stressed out mess, desperate to fix the situation. *What was wrong?* Did we have bad genes or was it something in the environment? We needed answers—so I started reading and researching again.

Eventually, my husband and I decided that we would try to avoid drugs, at least initially. We found some online information involving special diets and healing, which became the starting point for our diet adventure: an extended excursion into nutrition, gut-brain connections, friendly bacteria and the immune system.

Our first stop was probiotics. Not seeing much of an effect, we moved on to organic foods and then low carbohydrates. Our low carb diet included meats, eggs, yoghurt, homemade kefir, nuts, cheese, vegetables, fruits and honey. We brought nut cakes to birthday parties, making sure we were always prepared—it was *not easy*! The results?

(a) Jackie, our now three-year-old suddenly put the right words together, speaking in sentences. *What?! She could talk!*

(b) Emily, our eleven-year-old stopped sleepwalking almost immediately! *What a relief!*

These results were truly encouraging, signaling that with patience and hard work our kids would be able to recover. But the biggest reality check occurred in the back of my mind: if a simple diet change could have such profound effects—and we had been able to figure it out on our own—then why was our doctor in the dark about this information, in fact *why was it not on the evening news?*

I started reading every book about gut flora, researching the impact of beneficial bacteria, probiotic supplements and gut imbalances. My husband and I prepared fermented foods like kefir, kombucha and pickled cucumbers. I attended a debate, listening to the two sides discuss raw milk versus pasteurized milk,[1] and audience members declaring raw milk a miracle cure for their baby's eczema—*interesting!* We fermented soy beans into Japanese natto because it contained a special soil bacterium, deemed beneficial for a damaged gut. We cooked soups every day. I studied lactose and gluten intolerance, researching why some people can't handle them. It turned out that—in an unexpected twist—most of the fibers we eat were converted into fat by beneficial bacteria. S*o much for the no-fat salad dressing!* This explained how large cows could sustain themselves on a grass diet: by feeding green fibers to their stomach bacteria, they created a fermented sludge full of nutrients.

Optimum health could only occur if our intestines contained a healthy mix of beneficial bacteria, distributed from the mouth opening, through the stomach, and all the way down to the other exit. Every section of the digestive tract had its own group of friendly and helpful residents—each being affected by certain drugs, such as antibiotics, acid blockers and even birth control pills.[2] [3] I realized that it had been a mistake to take acid blockers for as long as I did because, by raising the pH in the stomach, they had prevented me from properly digesting protein foods. Most likely, they were also responsible for my bacterial overgrowth symptoms by allowing proliferation of the wrong organisms. In fact, the most likely explanation for my chronic stomach pain was probably an infection associated with *low* stomach acid, resulting in painful reflux.

The science of gut bacteria, also called microbiomics, explains

---

[1] Weston A. Price Foundation (WAPF), westonaprice.org

[2] Khalili, H. Risk of Inflammatory Bowel Disease with Oral Contraceptives and Menopausal Hormone Therapy: Current Evidence and Future Directions *Drug Saf.* **2016**, *39(3)*:193-197

[3] Skovlund, C.W. et al. Association of Hormonal Contraception With Depression JAMA Psychiatry, **2016**, *73(11)*:1154-1162

how harmful microorganisms like Clostridium difficile (C. diff) can generate toxins. Toxins which, when dominating the environment in the intestines, can even cause mental and emotional difficulties. Bloating, intestinal pain, poor concentration, anxiety and depression are likely related to microbiome imbalances. I found rumors about defective gut flora fermenting carbohydrates into alcohol—making people permanently drunk!

The rapidly developing field of microbiomics has blossomed into a new and well-respected branch of medical research with its own conferences and publications. There are now over 1000 books on Amazon, dealing in one form or another with low-carb nutrition and/or gut flora and healing through diet.

To sum up our nutritional adventures: healing through diet is a clear possibility, even when following a very basic plan. For us, low carbohydrates and probiotic foods worked wonders—there was a clearly noticeable change in the behaviors and abilities of our children! Picking a more complicated elimination diet might have been helpful under other circumstances; there is no one-size-fits-all.

And to anyone claiming that diet has no influence on illness, including mental/emotional ones—it's time for some homework, you need to catch up with facts! Worse yet, there are too many doctors ignoring new research which is staring them straight in the face. Healthcare providers desperately need to include some of this information in their patients' treatment plans!

In the end though, one question has stayed unanswered—what had been the reason for all our health problems in the first place? *What was at the root of it all?*

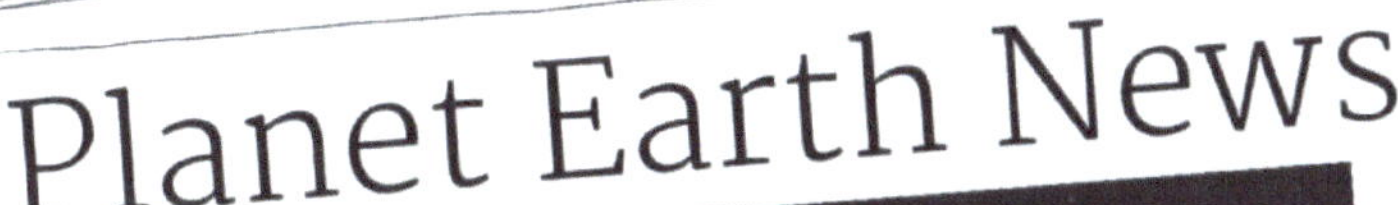

New Diet Concepts

from low-fat to paleo and back: a diet adventure with Lena Kratz

Details of the interview on page 10

My Personal Story:

Remarkable stories of healing food allergies, diabetes, depression eczema and autism.

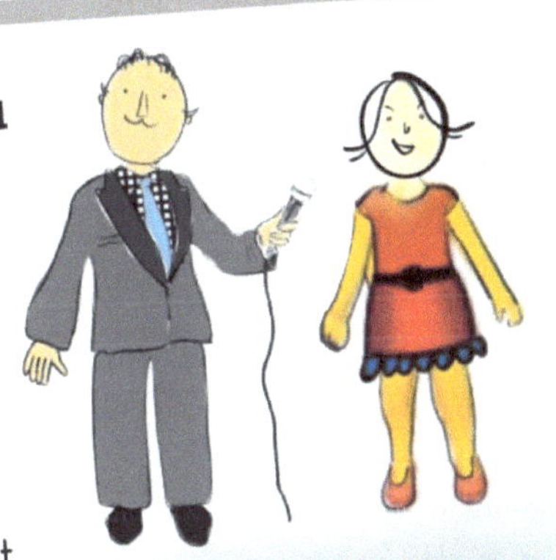

How To Heal Your Gut

Diet and Health. Diet and Health. Diet and Health.

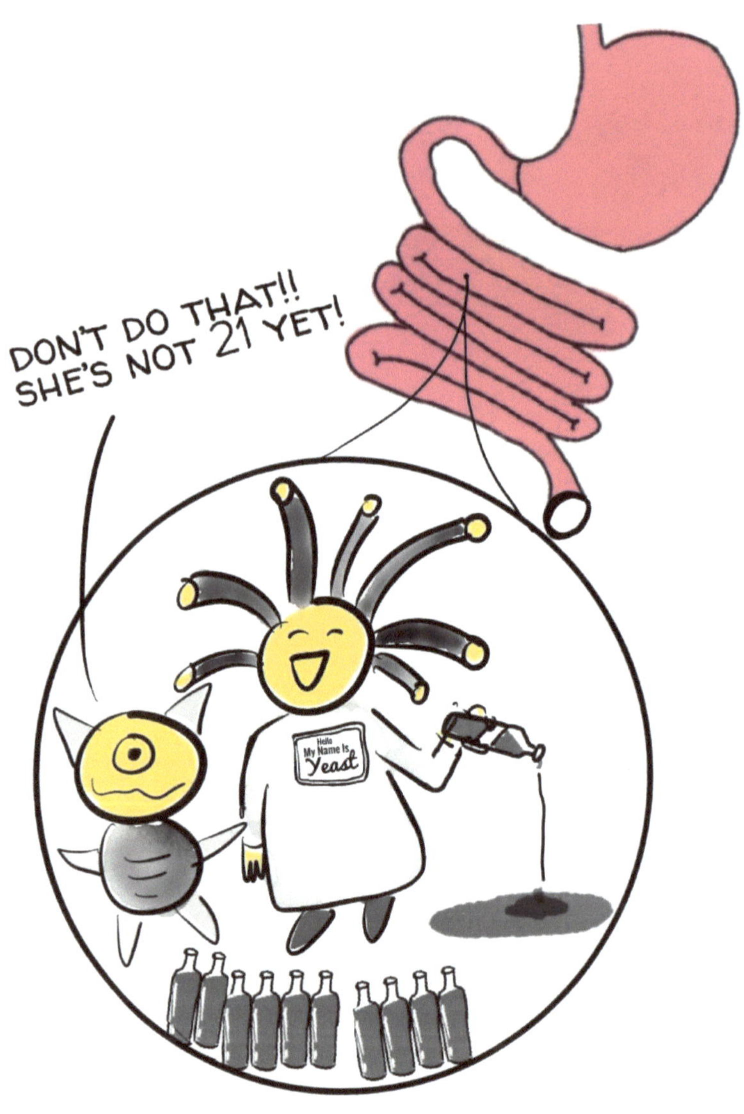
DON'T DO THAT!!
SHE'S NOT 21 YET!
Hello
My Name Is
Yeast

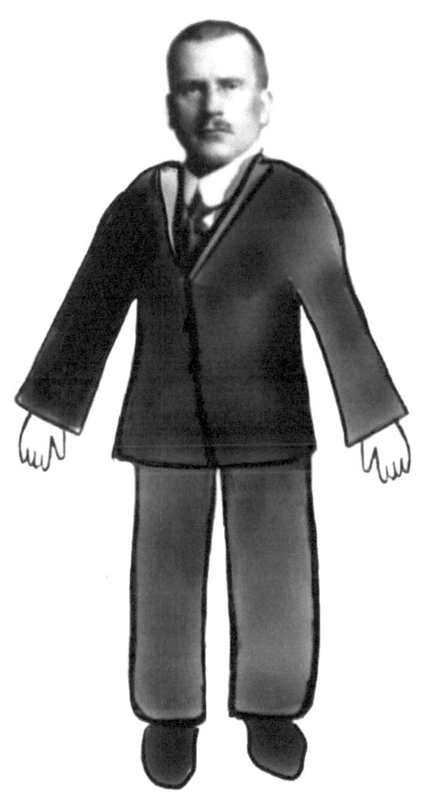

Carl Jung leaving Switzerland…

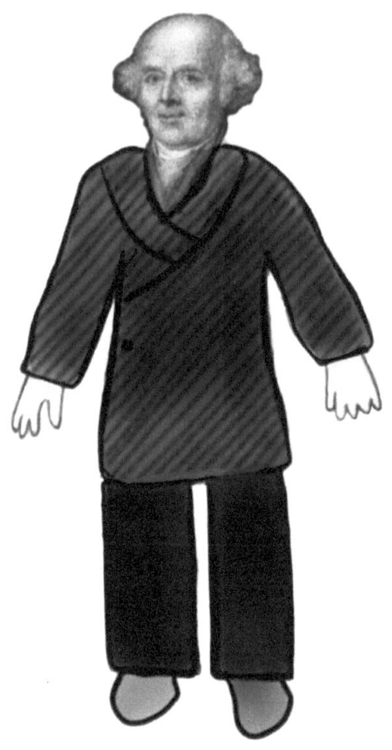

Samuel Hahnemann leaving Germany…

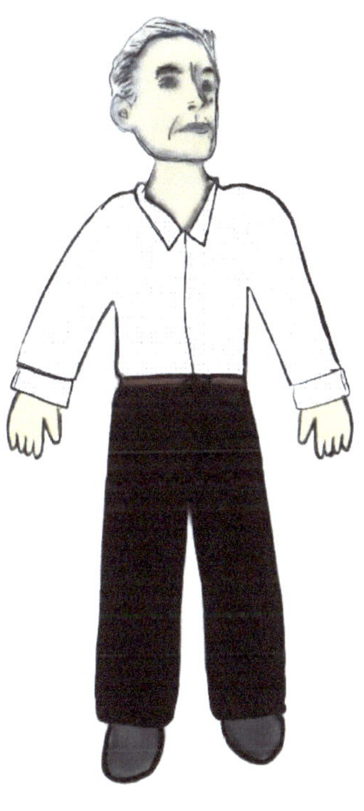

Jordan Peterson leaving Canada…

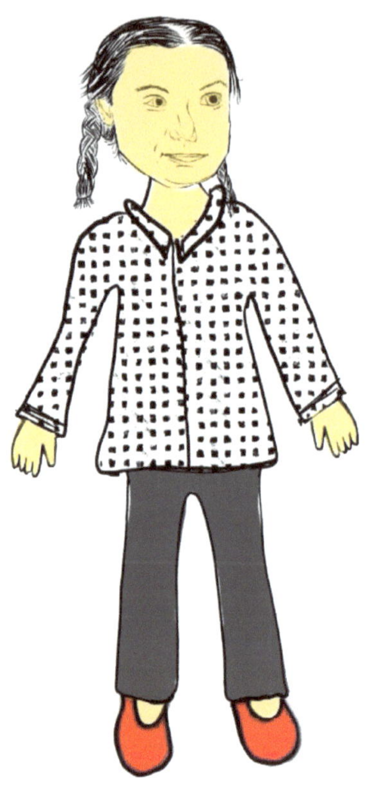

Greta Thunberg leaving Sweden…

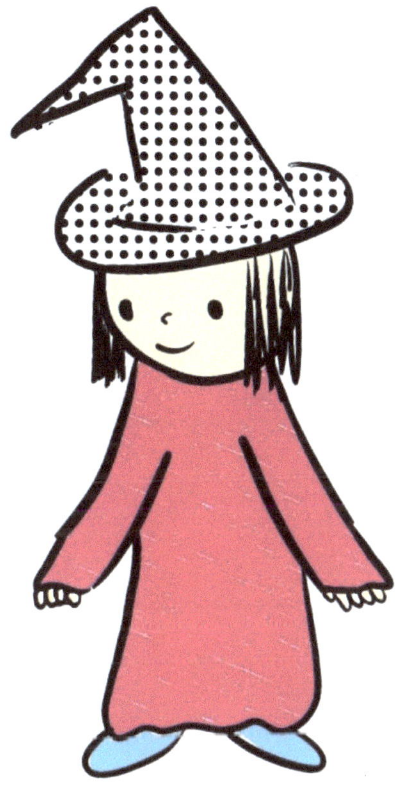

The Devouring Mother leaving somewhere…

Planet Earth News

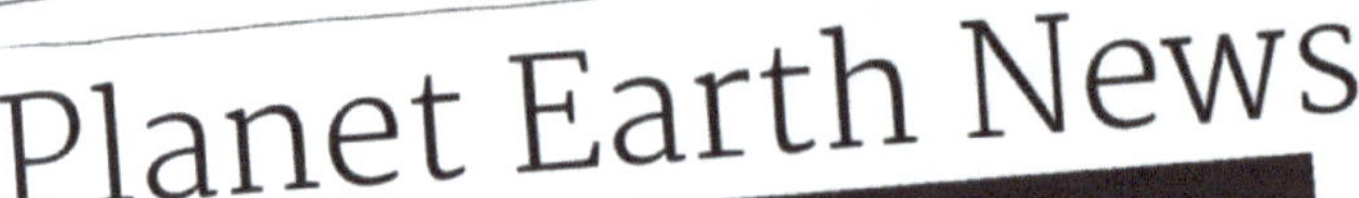

Weekend Edition: Party at Mother Nature's House! Full Report On Page 9

Exclusive: Who is invited?

Guest List a Secret

* * * * * * * * * * * * * * *

Mother Nature in her own words: "...good discussions and brainstorming..."

thinking about the future thinking about the future
thinking about the future thinking about the future

Secret Glimpse At Invitation!

please join us for
Food, Fun & Friends
Save The World!
at the Mother Nature Residency
Saturday 4:00pm
Planet Earth
Rsvp before July

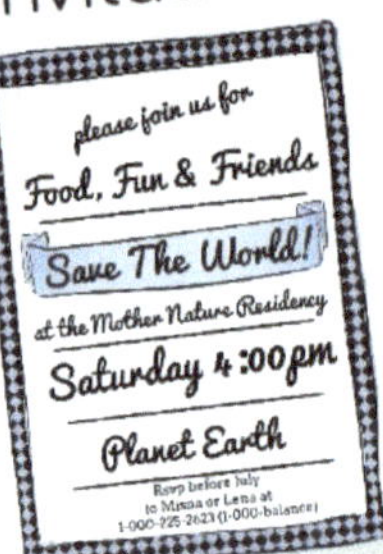

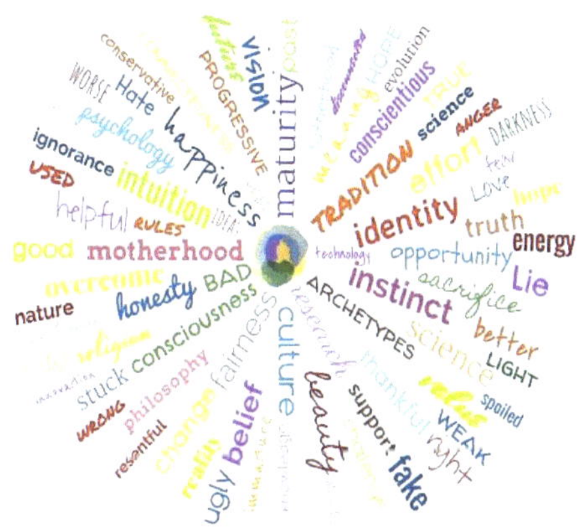
conservative
WORSE
Hate
psychology
happiness
PROGRESSIVE
vision
maturity
past
evolution
conscientious
science
ANGER
DARKNESS
TRADITION
effort
Love
ignorance
USED
intuition
helpful
RULES
identity
truth
energy
good
motherhood
technology
opportunity
Lie
instinct
sacrifice
honesty
BAD
nature
consciousness
ARCHETYPES
culture
better
science
LIGHT
stuck
philosophy
fairness
research
beauty
support
spoiled
WEAK
WRONG
resentful
change
belief
ugly
right
fake

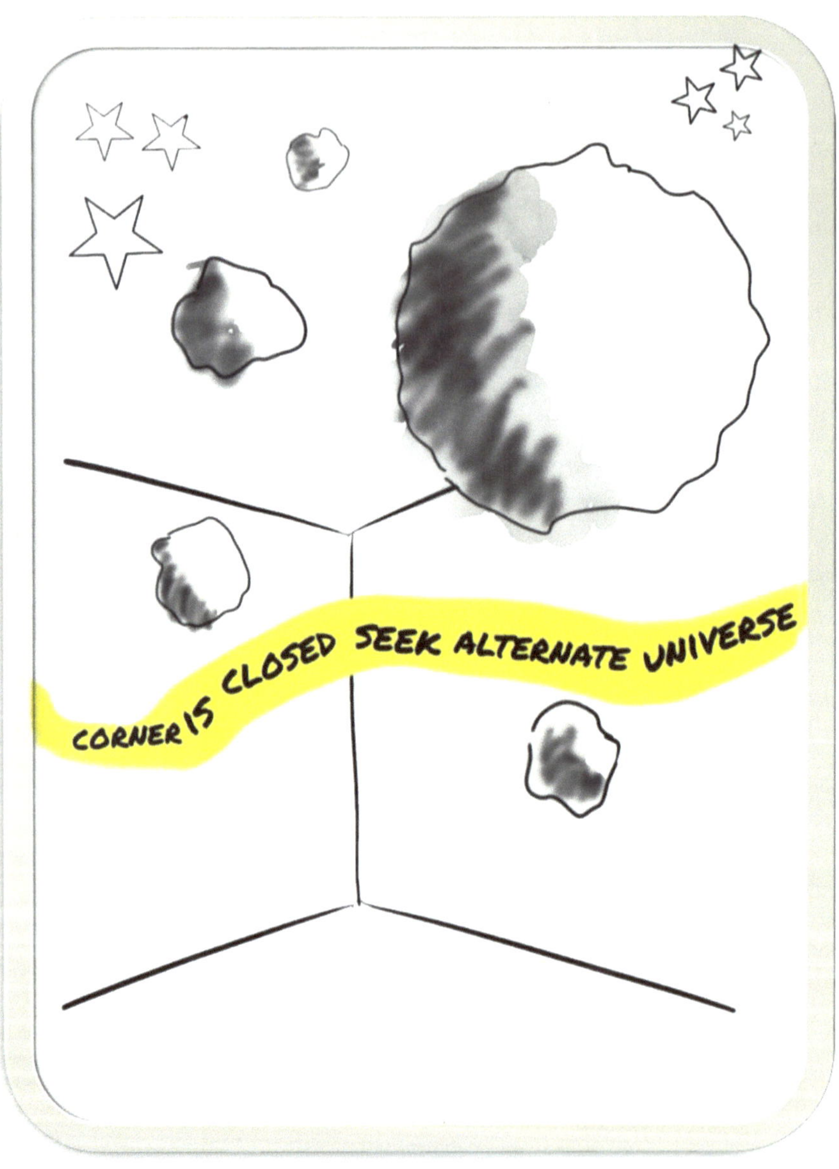
CORNER IS CLOSED SEEK ALTERNATE UNIVERSE

Forbidden Corners of the Universe

By Lena Kratz

I liked the diet, but then we reached a plateau. No matter how strict we were with our nutritional regime, we could not get to complete elimination of symptoms, limiting further healing. At night, we were punished for any transgressions when the old ailment came back. And yes, we could have chosen to be stricter, eliminating even more foods—*maybe that would have helped?* But then we learned that perhaps too strict of a low carb diet wasn't for everyone. Even though there were plenty of examples of human populations thriving in areas with naturally limited plant growth—relying exclusively on low carb animal foods—there had been examples of certain people doing poorly on such a diet. The main culprit was the loss of vitamin C, giving rise to scurvy.[4]

It was our first confrontation with the common one-size-fits-all concept that is the standard in medicine today and an inkling of what was to come in the form of archetypes. I started to constantly check myself—was I one of the unlucky ones who couldn't thrive on a low-carb diet? Did my gums bleed more easily now when I brushed my teeth?

To make matters worse, Emily, our now twelve-year-old, lost patience, demanding to know "when we could return to eating more fun food". I had no answer to that: would we have to stick with low-carb all our lives? I recognized that soon enough she would be making some of her own decisions, dropping the diet and buying a bunch of candy—and most likely all those ugly sleeping symptoms would come right back.

We tried to think of other options—and stumbled across homeopathy on the internet. Not knowing anything about it, but having nothing to lose, we made an appointment with a practitioner, who selected remedies for our children according to the weirdest, most illogical rules we had ever seen! This was certainly *very different* from anything pharma or diet related! The practitioner warned us that our children might suffer through "aggravations" and that taking the remedy

---

[4] Perfecthealthdiet.com

might intensify some of their current symptoms. He wasn't too worried about special diets; instead, he was generally in favor of eating wholesome organic foods of all kinds. I have to admit that we were skeptical at first but—*surprise!* —Emily's sleepwalking problems resolved themselves after just one dose of the prescribed remedy, with or without dietary transgressions! I was speechless. Reluctantly, over a period of a couple of weeks, we dropped the diet—and everything was fine! *Wow!*

We were impressed, returning to the practitioner to have remedies selected for ourselves. My acid stomach improved slowly but noticeably, and Jackie, our "delayed but improved" speaker thrived, turning from shy and introverted to talkative and outgoing. Suddenly, her interest in exploring the world exploded, she kept touching everything while asking a million questions—all within a couple of months!

Six months later, she had taught herself to read, ready for kindergarten. For my husband it took longer to see real progress, and we learned that if the remedy was mismatched, there would be no improvement. Good outcomes depended on a combination of three things: the clarity of symptoms, the severity of the case and the competence of the practitioner.

With these drawbacks in mind, we became regular homeopathy clients, observing many positive changes during this time. Improvements in attitude were common—an unexpected bonus no other medical treatment had ever delivered as a byproduct. I gratefully acknowledged this positive change in emotional state, noticing that it usually came hand in hand with a shift in physical symptoms.

The whole experience had been so out of the blue—so bewildering—I wondered how I had missed this side of medical care for so many years. Why wasn't it more popular? Why had no one ever talked about it in school, during work or at parties? It was puzzling.

But deep down I knew why it wasn't more widespread. It was the suspiciously arbitrary guessing procedure of remedy selection, confusing people and making practitioners look like spirit healers rather than health consultants or scientists. Clearly, there had to be more to it, and I was determined to find out, so my husband and I set out to study homeopathy. By fall of that year we were enrolled in our first classes.

Considering that we had spent our whole lives around mainstream science, this was a pretty big jump for us. No other scientists were out there—at least not many—looking at these forbidden corners of the universe. We were happy when we found one: former NASA scientist Amy Lansky who had come across homeopathy while looking for solutions to improve her son's autism. The admittedly provocative title of her book *Impossible Cure* chronicles her experiences and treatment choices. [5] It is a great book—every time I am asked to explain homeopathy, I recommend her book as an introduction.

We realized that learning homeopathy wasn't going to be easy. The material was completely different from chemistry, difficult in a new and uncommon way, never seen before. This was no wishy-washy obscure theory; in fact, the opposite was true—it had a solid scientific base of understanding behind it, created two hundred years ago in Germany by medical doctor and scientist Dr. Samuel Hahnemann. All it required was some rethinking.[6]

After a few lessons the most important point turned out to be this: diseases were groups of symptoms occurring on three planes—a physical, an emotional and a mental plane. These three planes all contributed to an image of a person which was to be matched with a similar remedy picture. The picture consisted of more than just a collection of common symptoms thrown together in a pile; instead, it was rather specific. It was, in fact, so specific that it included a whole range of personality traits—from favorite foods and preferences in clothing to attitudes about work, family or fun things to do on a weekend. In other words: remedy selection was based on archetypes.[7]

---

[5] Lansky, A. *Impossible Cure*, R.L.Ranch Press, **2003**

[6] Vithoulkas, G. *The Science of Homeopathy*, Grove Weidenfeld, **1980**

[7] Coulter, C.R. *Nature and Human Personality: Homeopathic Archetypes*, Ninth House Publishing, West Virginia, **2002**

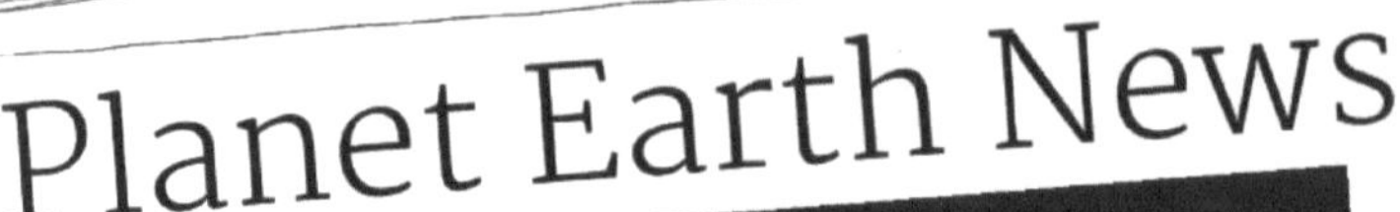
Planet Earth News
Hahnemann On Moving To Paris: All On Track
How come I haven't heard of it? 200 year old research makes comeback! go to page 8 for details
What is the vital force? page 5
Our experts provide an answer
Hahnemann excited about party: "love stimulating discussions, meeting people I disagree with..."
Exclusive summary on page 12

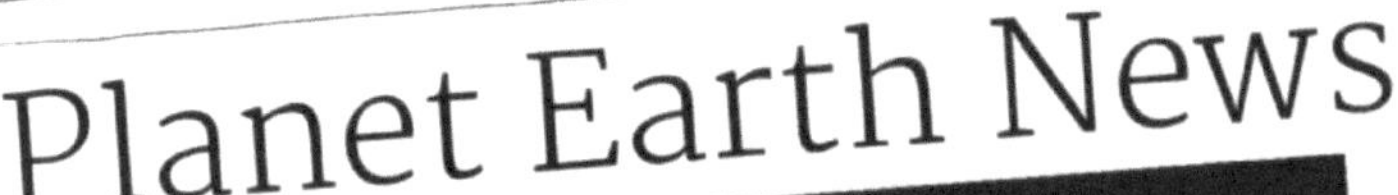

Planet Earth News

Exclusive: Plane Review
Which Plane Is Best?
Immune System Engineers
Answer Your Questions

Samuel Hahnemann on why the physical plane is best exclusive details on page 5

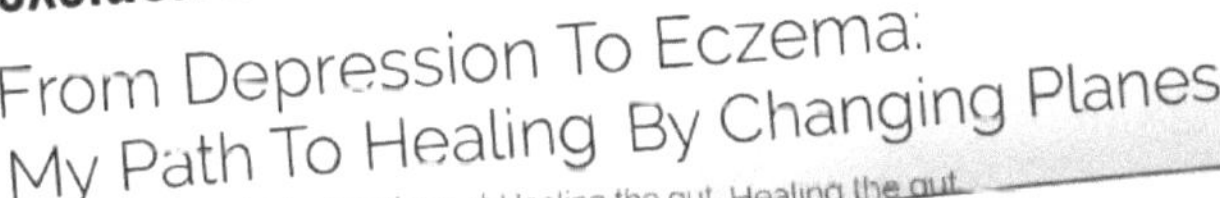

From Depression To Eczema:
My Path To Healing By Changing Planes

Healing the gut Healing the gut Healing the gut Healing the gut

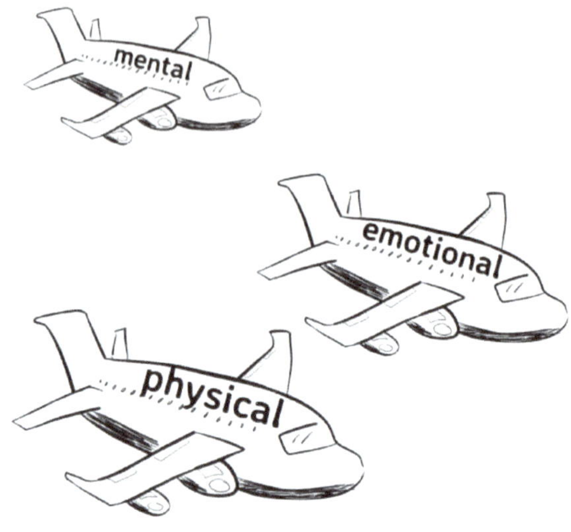
mental
emotional
physical

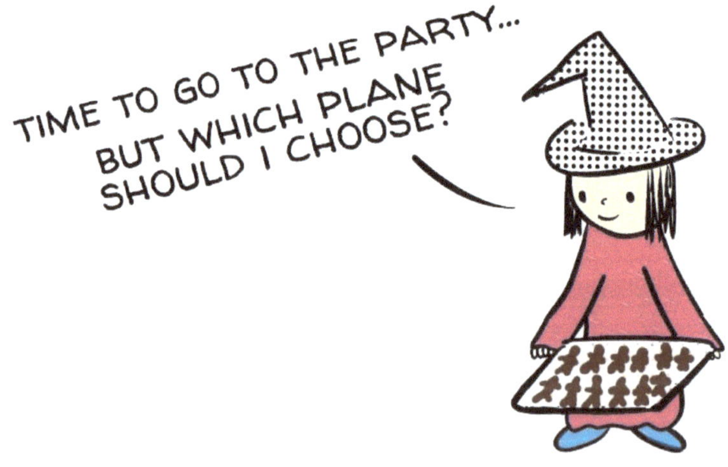
TIME TO GO TO THE PARTY...
BUT WHICH PLANE
SHOULD I CHOOSE?

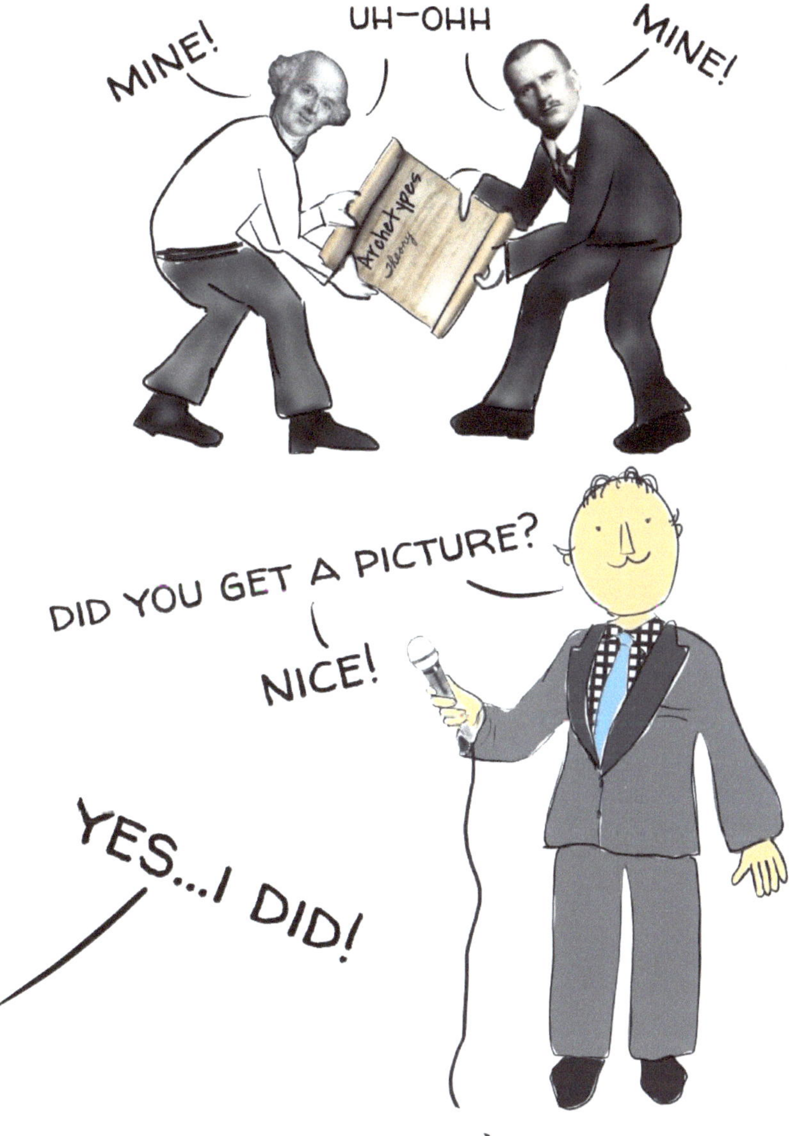
MINE!
UH-OHH
MINE!
Archetypes
theory
DID YOU GET A PICTURE?
NICE!
YES...I DID!

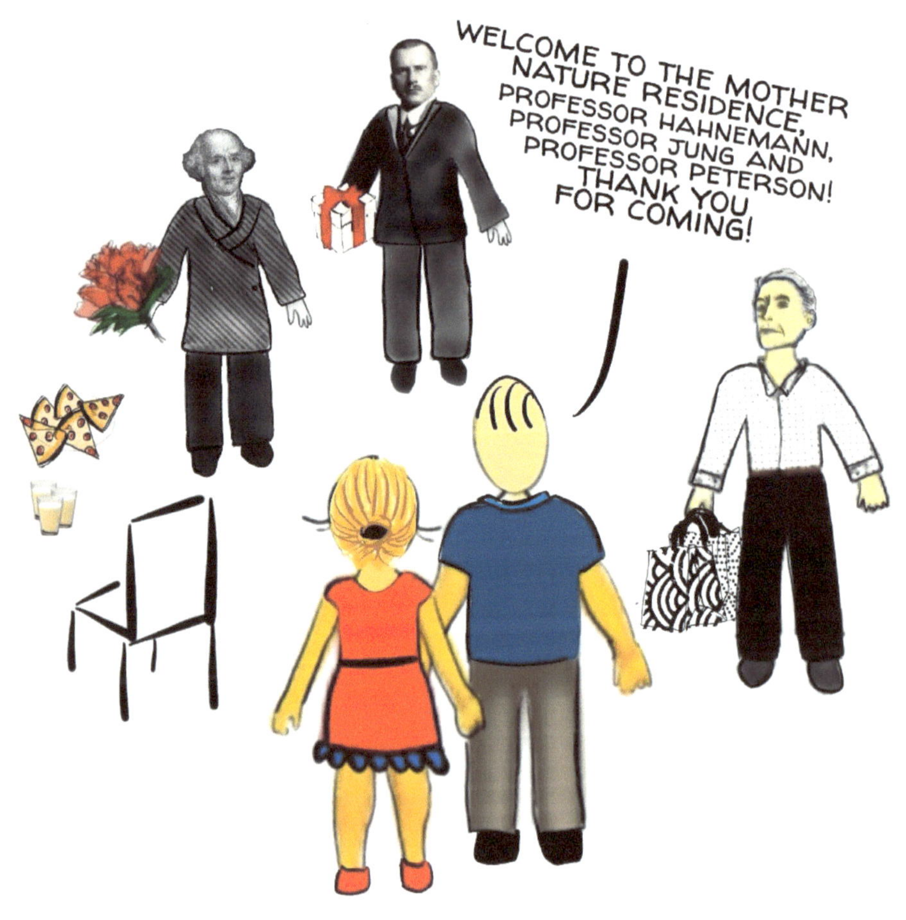
WELCOME TO THE MOTHER NATURE RESIDENCE, PROFESSOR HAHNEMANN, PROFESSOR JUNG AND PROFESSOR PETERSON! THANK YOU FOR COMING!

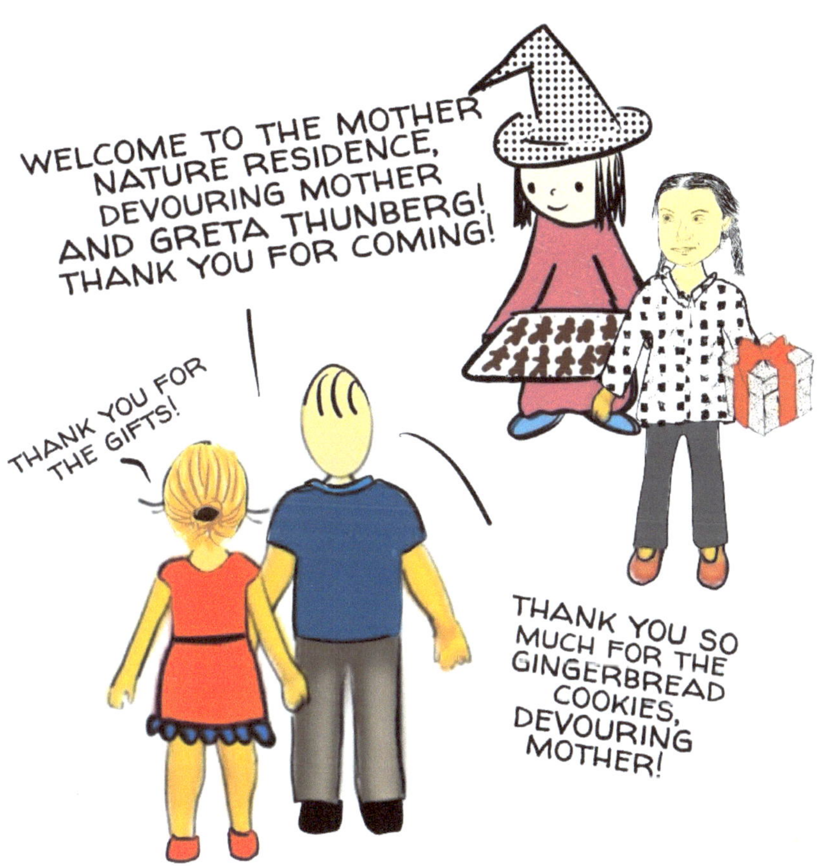
WELCOME TO THE MOTHER NATURE RESIDENCE, DEVOURING MOTHER AND GRETA THUNBERG! THANK YOU FOR COMING!
THANK YOU FOR THE GIFTS!
THANK YOU SO MUCH FOR THE GINGERBREAD COOKIES, DEVOURING MOTHER!

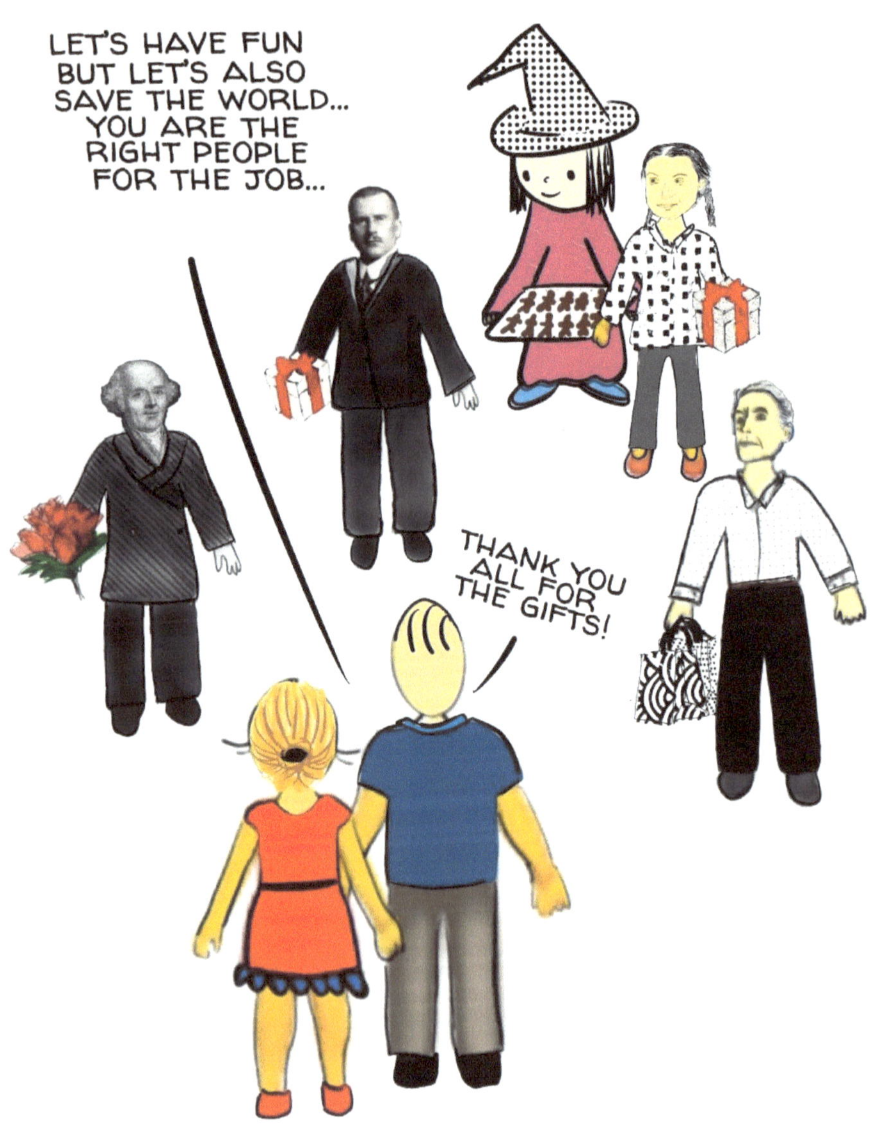
LET'S HAVE FUN
BUT LET'S ALSO
SAVE THE WORLD...
YOU ARE THE
RIGHT PEOPLE
FOR THE JOB...
THANK YOU
ALL FOR
THE GIFTS!

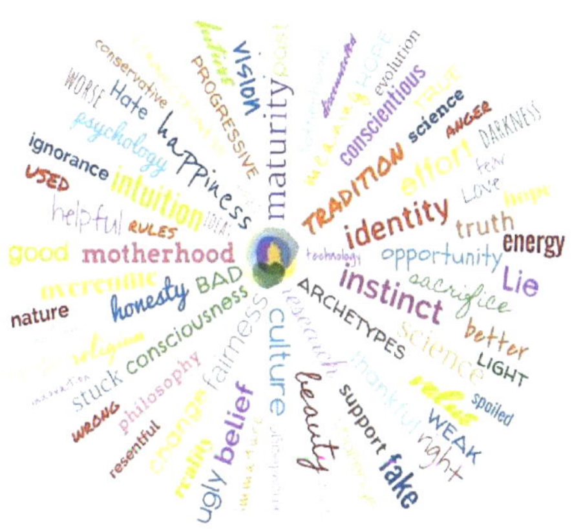
maturity
identity
motherhood
instinct
culture
intuition
happiness
honesty
consciousness
opportunity
TRADITION
conscientious
science
effort
truth
energy
Lie
sacrifice
better
LIGHT
spoiled
WEAK
fake
support
beauty
belief
ugly
change
philosophy
resentful
WRONG
stuck
nature
good
helpful
RULES
USED
ignorance
psychology
Hate
WORSE
conservative
PROGRESSIVE
VISION
evolution
ANGER
DARKNESS
Love
fairness
BAD
ARCHETYPES
technology
IDEAS

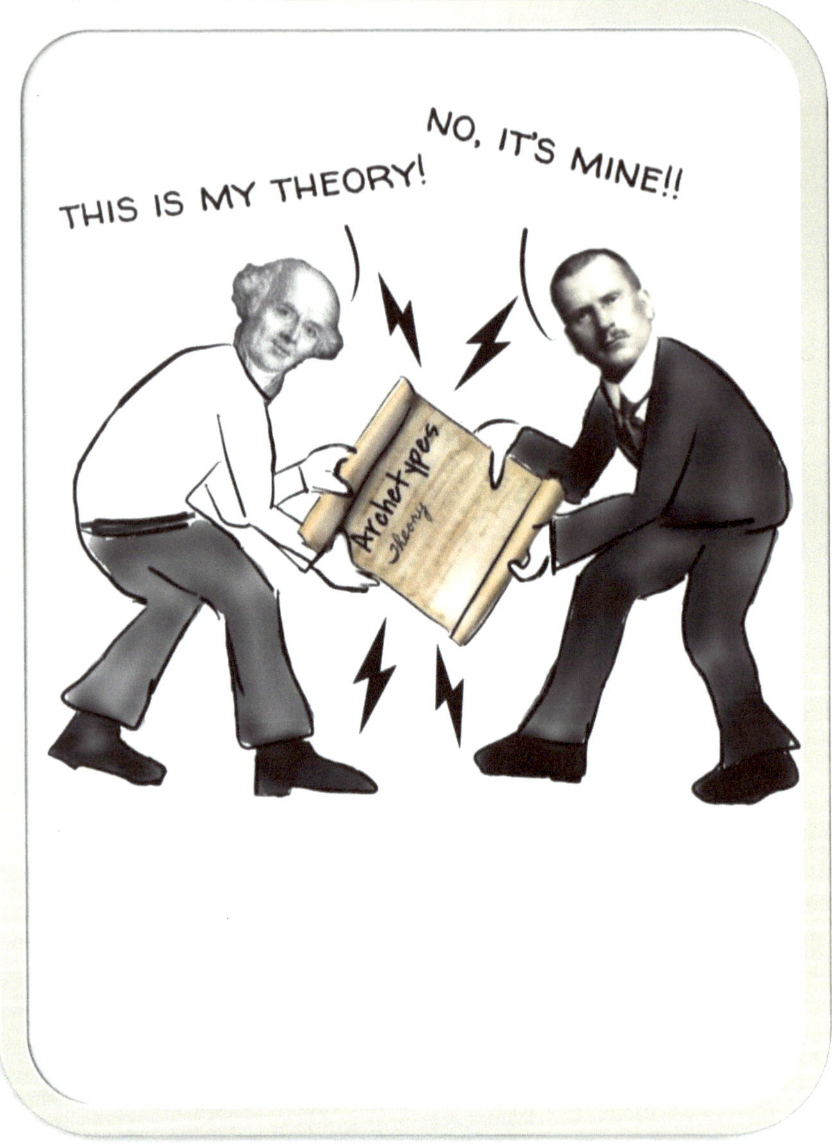
THIS IS MY THEORY!
NO, IT'S MINE!!
Archetypes
theory

The Archetypes

By Misna Burelli

What are archetypes? The word archetype is derived from the Greek word "arkhetupon", which roughly means "original pattern". Generally speaking, an archetype is a character model or standard example, similar to a prototype, explaining concepts that are typical for a variety of situations.

Good, recognizable archetypes are like universal patterns, appearing as representative characters in stories throughout history.[8] The human mind seems to be drawn towards these tales representing universal truths—they sound strangely familiar. Most of us intuitively resonate with characters that fit expected archetypes, but not with others, who appear inauthentic.[9] [10]

A number of people have studied archetypes, but one of the most famous scholars to contend with the topic was Carl Jung (1875-1961), a Swiss psychiatrist and professor, who developed a theory of the collective unconscious as the basis for his Jungian archetypes.[11] The concept has recently been revived in the public sphere by Jordan Peterson,[12] himself a well-known clinical psychologist and professor of psychology from Canada. Calling himself a Jungian analyst, his writings reflect much of the same culture-analytical style that characterized Jung's work.

Many people are probably more familiar with the commonly applied Myers-Briggs personality indicator, as the test is often a part of company sponsored employee training.[13] It sorts individuals into sixteen personality categories, making it possible to analyze potential managerial styles, team compatibility, and creative vision. Among the choices are:

---

[8] Booker, C. *The Seven Basic Plots: Why We Tell Stories*, London, Continuum **2006**
[9] Van Bergen, J. *Archetypes for Writers: Using the Power of Your Subconscious* Michael Wiese Productions, **2007**
[10] Rosenfeld, J. *Make a Scene*, Writer's Digest Books, **2017**
[11] Jung, C. *Man and His Symbols*, Dell Publishing Co., Inc. **1968**
[12] https://www.jordanbpeterson.com
[13] The Myers&Briggs Foundation at https://www.myersbriggs.org

extroverts/introverts (E/I), thinkers/feelers (T/F), sensors/intuitives (S/I), and judgers/perceivers (J/P).[14] The resulting four letters describe you as one of the sixteen (4x4) variations that are possible under the Myers-Briggs rules. These sixteen repeating patterns—archetypes—distinguish between certain personalities, while grouping others together. The Myers-Briggs test relies solely on psychological markers without including any physical attributes.

No matter which theory one follows, such a categorization process is usually performed in a psychoanalytical manner, helping with self-awareness to overcome past trauma, or as a springboard for personal or career development. Archetype categories are also often used in marketing research. [15]

Jung was not the first to spot some of these repeating human character patterns. A number of researchers have noticed that people are often both unique and alike. [16] [17] In fact, the beginnings of this theory go all the way back to Plato, Kant, Schopenhauer,[18] and, of course, Samuel Hahnemann. Hahnemann (1755-1843) found a whole range of human archetypes, many more than just sixteen! Hahnemann's and Jung's theories overlap, with no evidence of the succeeding Jung being aware of Hahnemann or applying Hahnemann's ideas in his own research.

So, let's assume that it's true—that we can sort all humans into archetypal groups—by means of personality traits, psychological qualities, and perhaps even physical characteristics. That sounds reasonable enough—why don't we just pick our favorite theory and start categorizing ourselves? It could be interesting, except for one problem: whose theory is correct? What is a recognizable archetype? Hypotheses about belonging to one versus another personality category have been ample; as mentioned earlier, it appears that every scholar has made up

---

[14] http://www.humanmetrics.com/personality/type

[15] *Retail therapy. How Ernest Dichter, an acolyte of Sigmund Freud, revolutionized marketing* The Economist, Dec 17, **2011**

[16] Odajnyk, V. *Archetype and Character: Power, Eros, Spirit, and Matter Personality Types*, Palgrave Macmillan, **2012**

[17] Holtkamp, M.B. *Biology of the Archetype*, Mark Holtkamp, **2014**

[18] Jung CG, Letters Vol. II, p. 500-502

their own personal archetype collection. Sometimes there is overlap between researchers and other times not, leading to the suspicion that much of their work is based on opinions, rather than strict scientific rules. All theories are based on their own unique classification criteria, with their own advantages and drawbacks, rather than focusing on universal truths. Sure, there are similarities, bringing some models closer together than others, but none of them resemble a script grounded in logical rules. So, how do we sort it out? For archetypes to be useful at all, the observed traits have to be common enough to form a group, validating their importance. Focusing on such common data points creates a framework for analyzing potential archetypes in an array of otherwise irrelevant noise. Most theories start out with basic, well-accepted, easily distinguishable psychological group identity traits: outgoing, quiet, shy, friendly, jealous, aggressive, compassionate, creative, oversensitive, passionate, driven, weak, sneaky, mean—they could all be used to categorize people.

Depending on how detailed the classification is supposed to become, we can include more such qualities—the list could go on and on. At first, we will see a general personal baseline emerge, changing into a more detailed picture, and as more data points are collected, they transform again into a comprehensive description of a real human being. Just like in the art world—the more data points we collect, the higher the resolution of the resulting picture.

But in the end, it always leads to the same problem: how much resolution do we need to define a "true" category? There are no clear standards. There are no preferred rules. Should men and woman be separated? Are the attempts— debated by Jung and Peterson—to classify certain traits as "feminine chaos" versus "masculine order" a valid distinction or not? What is a genuine archetype, as opposed to a separate entity due to biological makeup, species, or gender differences?

We won't be able to solve this puzzle unless we are able to find truly *universal* patterns that cannot be shifted according to someone's point of view.

So how about this? We come up with a standard by collecting *all data!* Yes, that's right—all data, including all the physical, mental and emotional states humans have *ever* experienced. Sounds too hard? Not really! This is exactly what homeopaths have been doing for a couple of centuries! They collected all data, and that is the reason why homeopathic archetypes are *really detailed*, and where homeopathy is also *truly different* from all the other archetype theories. Of all the "personality tests" out there, the homeopathic one is *by far* the most comprehensive!

But Samuel Hahnemann, the inventor of homeopathy, went even one step further: he connected personality archetypes to remedy pictures. In other words, by basing the archetype on a combination of detailed personality characteristics and medically diagnosed disease symptoms, he was able to match the emerging picture with a natural substance, in the form of a remedy. By connecting the two, he created a *self-confirming* theory based on *natural laws.* As explained earlier, only the right remedy helps the body to heal, thereby automatically confirming archetype selection.[19]

When Hahnemann spoke of disease as a disturbance to the body of an organism, he recognized that there were dynamic influences outside the body, producing a "pathologically untuned vital force" (aphorisms 11 and 12, *Organon of Medicine*).[20] The degree of disturbance could be recognized by the "totality of symptoms on three planes". This is a Hahnemann specific term, indicating that *all symptoms* were supposed to be collected and analyzed—physical, mental and emotional ones.

Not much has changed since then; the homeopathic process has been the same for two hundred years. Homeopaths compare archetype images to known remedy pictures from a previously established database. Records for this database have been accumulated through experience, meticulously documenting successfully matched pictures, resulting in cures, and through a process called "proving". "Proving" is mistranslated from the German word "Prüfung", and actually means testing or checking. Considering that many homeopathic provings were carried out at a time before computer records were available, one can

---

[19] Remedy pictures are typically described in detail in a Materia Medica. There are many well-known Materia Medicas by different authors, some going back a couple of centuries

[20] Hahnemann, S. *Organon of Medicine,* Koethen, Germany, **1810**

imagine the monumental task of building such a database using mostly paper and pencil. Provings—still common today—have been performed in the exact same way for about two hundred years, forming a cornerstone of homeopathic research. New data are constantly added into this existing enormous database.

Earlier records were eventually transferred into books called repertories, which are still used and in print today, such as the classic Kent repertory.[21] These original repertories, and their modern versions, are great resources if you really want to learn about human behavior, associated archetypes and suffering—all kinds of suffering!

In the meantime, homeopaths have digitized many of the data, making archetype selection via computer a much less time-consuming endeavor.

You may wonder what kind of data we are talking about, generating mountains of files to be searched—and where they came from. This question has an easy answer: if you record *all symptoms* from an hour-long doctor's appointment, adding some past history and relevant family information, it will produce plenty of notes. And yes—doctor's appointments need to be longer than twenty minutes, which is exactly how homeopathic consultations are structured. These are not therapy sessions, but simply an attempt to collect the data of *all symptoms*. It is still done the exact same way today. If it feels like therapy to some, it's because collecting symptoms on all planes—mental, emotional and physical ones—and talking about them with your doctor actually often feels like therapy.

Because homeopathy has been around for about two hundred years, evolving and incorporating new information all the time, we know a lot about the most common remedies, like those for sale at various vitamin stores. These remedies have extremely well-known archetypes. We are able to truly describe their character, detailing a multitude of potential physical symptoms and emotions most commonly present, if applicable. And then there are other lesser known remedies, which are

---

[21] Kent, J.T. *Repertory of the Homeopathic Materia Medica*, B Jain Publishers (P) LTD. Sixth American Edition, **2009** (First American Edition: **1897)**

mostly used in complimentary fashions, or when common remedies do not apply. A third category of remedies, so called "nosodes", are made from disease materials, and thus are often used to help clear out these same specific diseases. Interestingly, the disease material remedies often carry archetype pictures corresponding to some of the cultural norms or concerns of the time of the disease outbreak. They are like historical archetypes, describing the Zeitgeist. Big epidemics like tuberculosis, syphilis, and gonorrhea, for example, influenced culture, leaving archetype imprints for generations to come. These imprints can be observed even today. In homeopathy, this is called a "miasm".

Under homeopathic theory, many people naturally tend toward one or several archetypes, and their corresponding remedies, throughout their life. This happens even without suffering from major disease symptoms, and the related remedies are called constitutional remedies. Often, the constitutional picture remains valid for years, if not decades, especially if there is a strong family history involving a particular archetype. Children are likely to retain some of the mother's or father's archetypes. Archetypes are not set in stone; they can often change or overlap with time. Environmental factors play an additional role, as do certain current communicable diseases and previous ones, affecting the ancestors on both sides of the family (miasm). We will be taking a look at the theory of miasms and suppression in later chapters.

Planet Earth News

Our Reporter On The Case: Embarrassing? Yes! But: Conflict Has Not Been Resolved! **go to page 11**

Caught On Camera:
Dr. Hahnemann and Dr. Jung in fist fight!

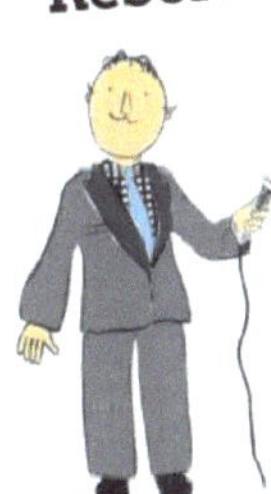

Both Researchers Claim Theory For Themselves!

What Theory?
Experts Weigh In

The Devouring Mother: each should get half a theory! commentary on page 7

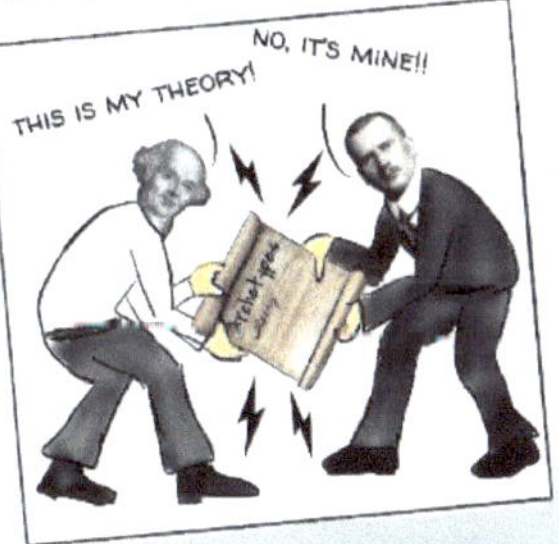

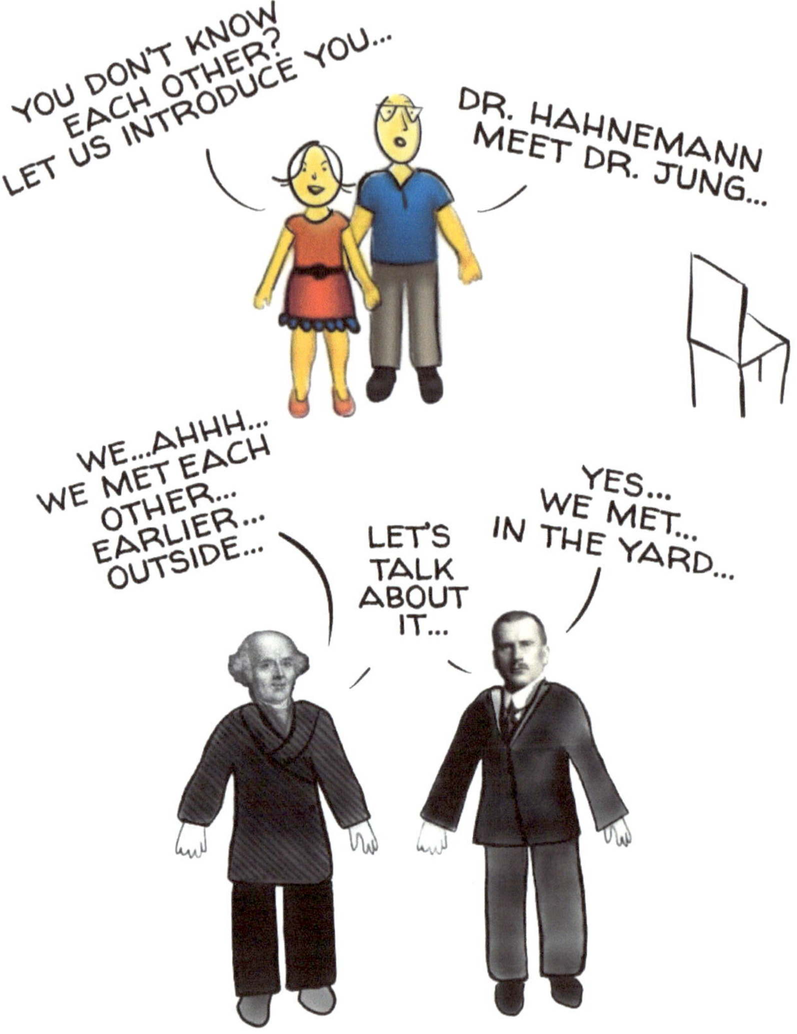
YOU DON'T KNOW EACH OTHER? LET US INTRODUCE YOU...
DR. HAHNEMANN MEET DR. JUNG...
WE...AHHH... WE MET EACH OTHER... EARLIER... OUTSIDE...
LET'S TALK ABOUT IT...
YES... WE MET... IN THE YARD...

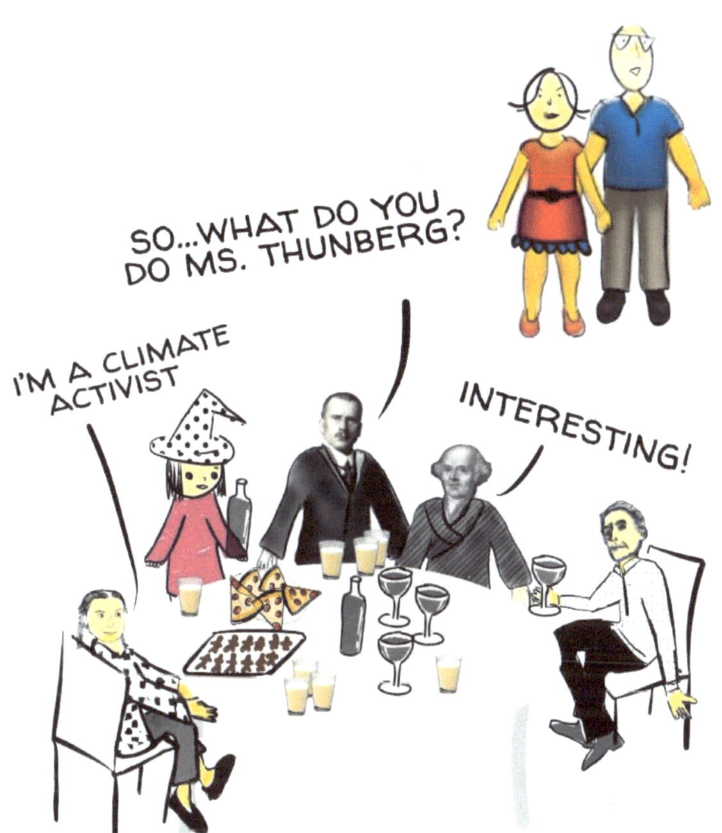
SO...WHAT DO YOU DO MS. THUNBERG?
I'M A CLIMATE ACTIVIST
INTERESTING!

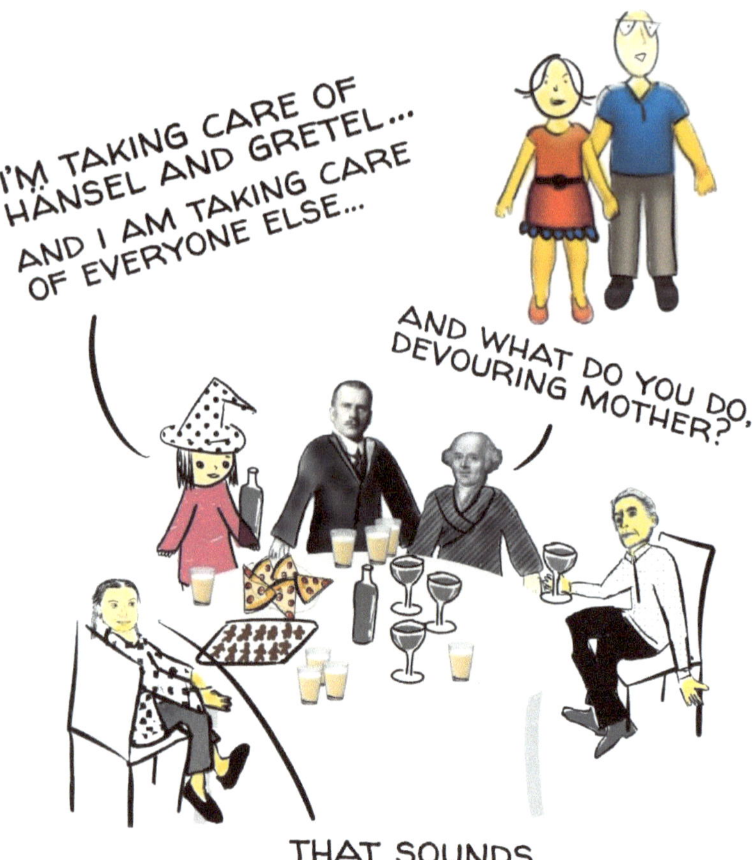
I'M TAKING CARE OF HÄNSEL AND GRETEL...
AND I AM TAKING CARE OF EVERYONE ELSE...
AND WHAT DO YOU DO, DEVOURING MOTHER?
THAT SOUNDS VERY NICE!

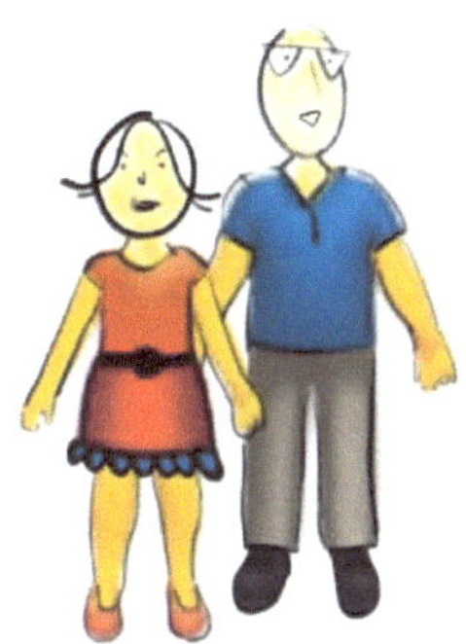

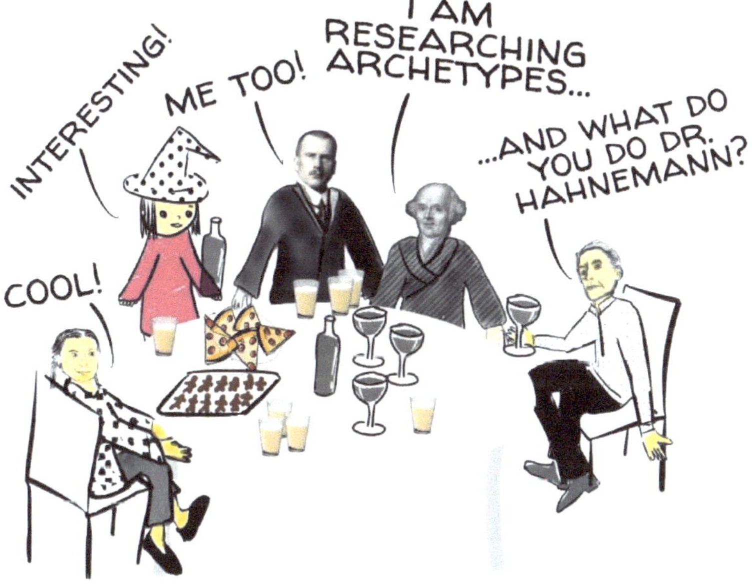
COOL!
INTERESTING!
ME TOO!
I AM RESEARCHING ARCHETYPES...
...AND WHAT DO YOU DO DR. HAHNEMANN?

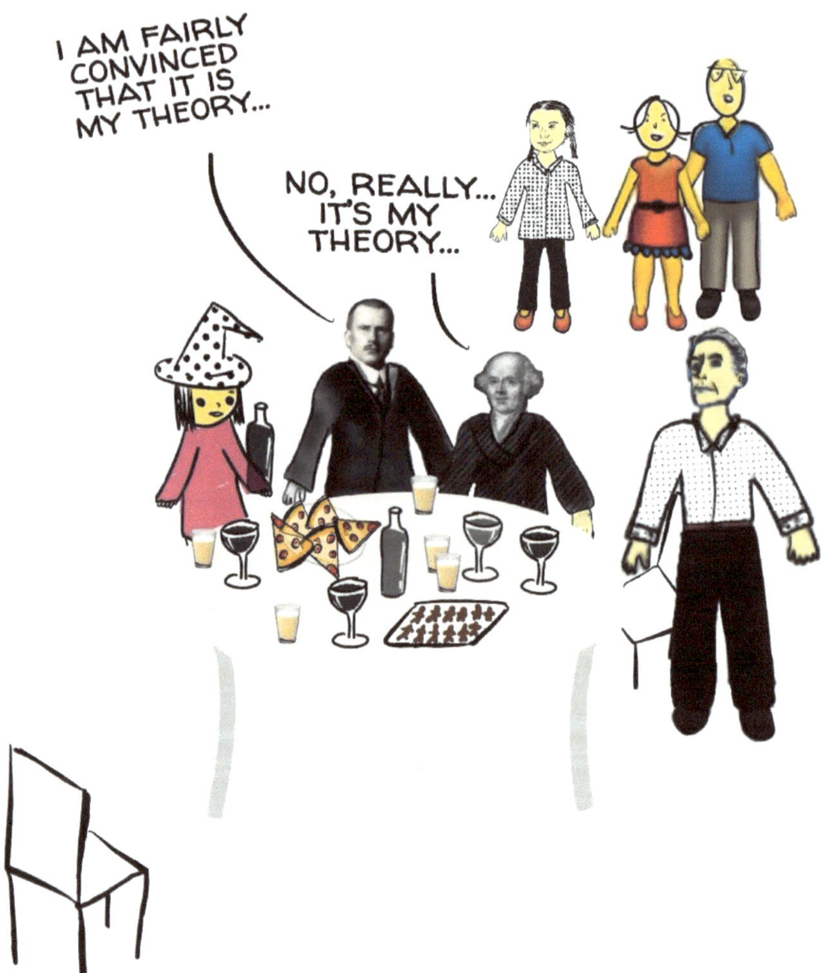
I AM FAIRLY CONVINCED THAT IT IS MY THEORY...
NO, REALLY... IT'S MY THEORY...

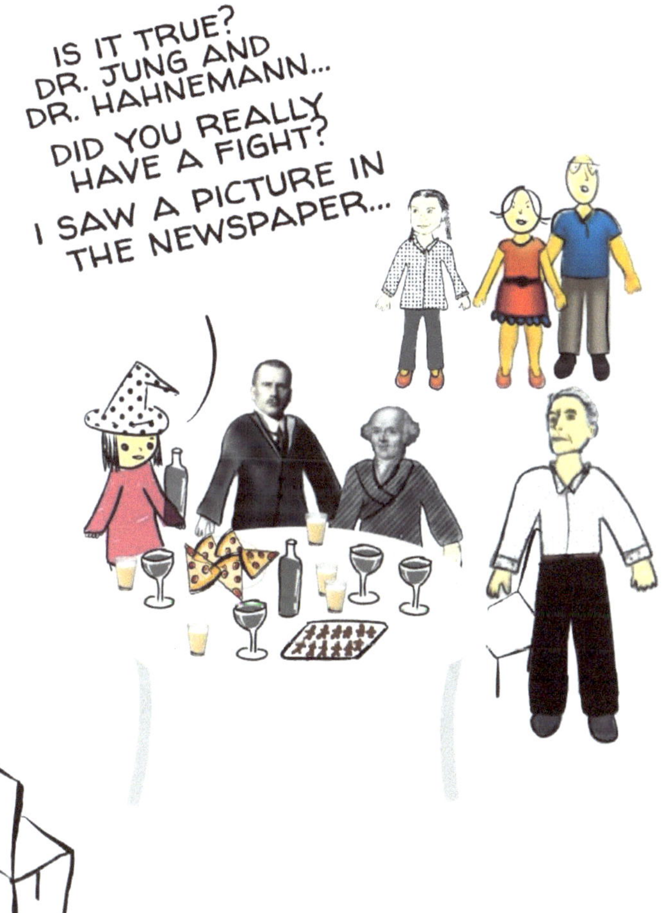
IS IT TRUE?
DR. JUNG AND
DR. HAHNEMANN...
DID YOU REALLY
HAVE A FIGHT?
I SAW A PICTURE IN
THE NEWSPAPER...

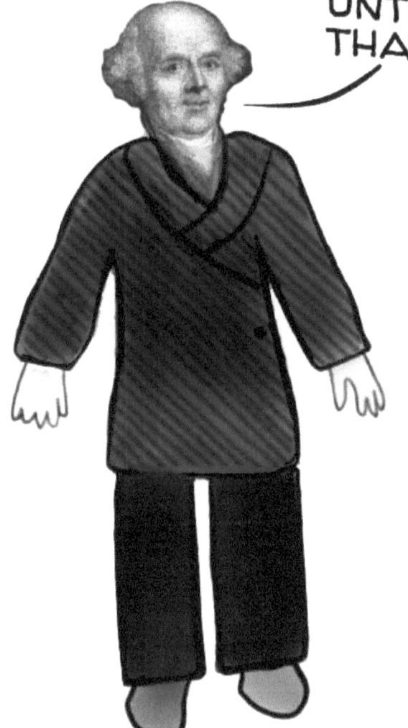
IT IS ONLY THE PATHOLOGICALLY UNTUNED VITAL FORCE THAT CAUSES DISEASE...

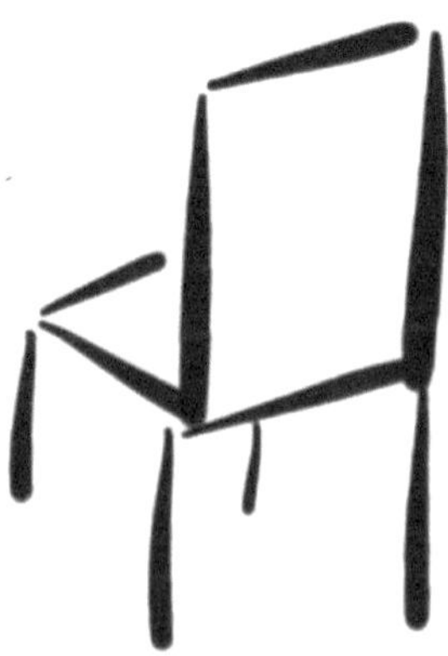

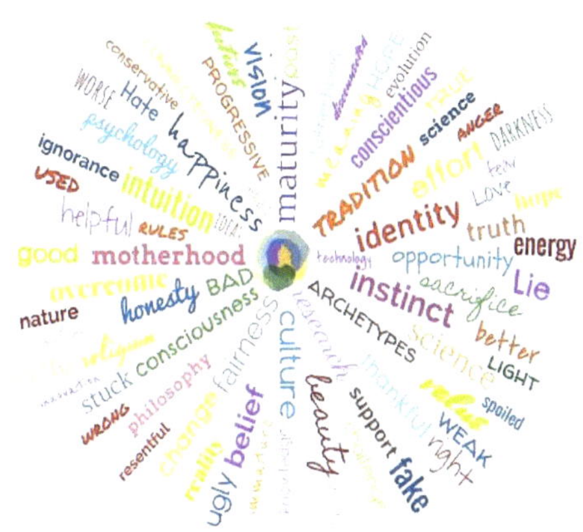
conservative
WORSE
Hate
PROGRESSIVE
VISION
maturity
evolution
conscientious
science
ANGER
DARKNESS
psychology
happiness
ignorance
USED
intuition
TRADITION
effort
LOVE
hope
helpful
RULES
identity
truth
energy
good
motherhood
technology
opportunity
sacrifice
Lie
honesty
BAD
instinct
nature
consciousness
ARCHETYPES
better
science
LIGHT
stuck
fairness
culture
research
philosophy
beauty
thankful
spoiled
WRONG
change
belief
support
WEAK
resentful
right
ugly
fake

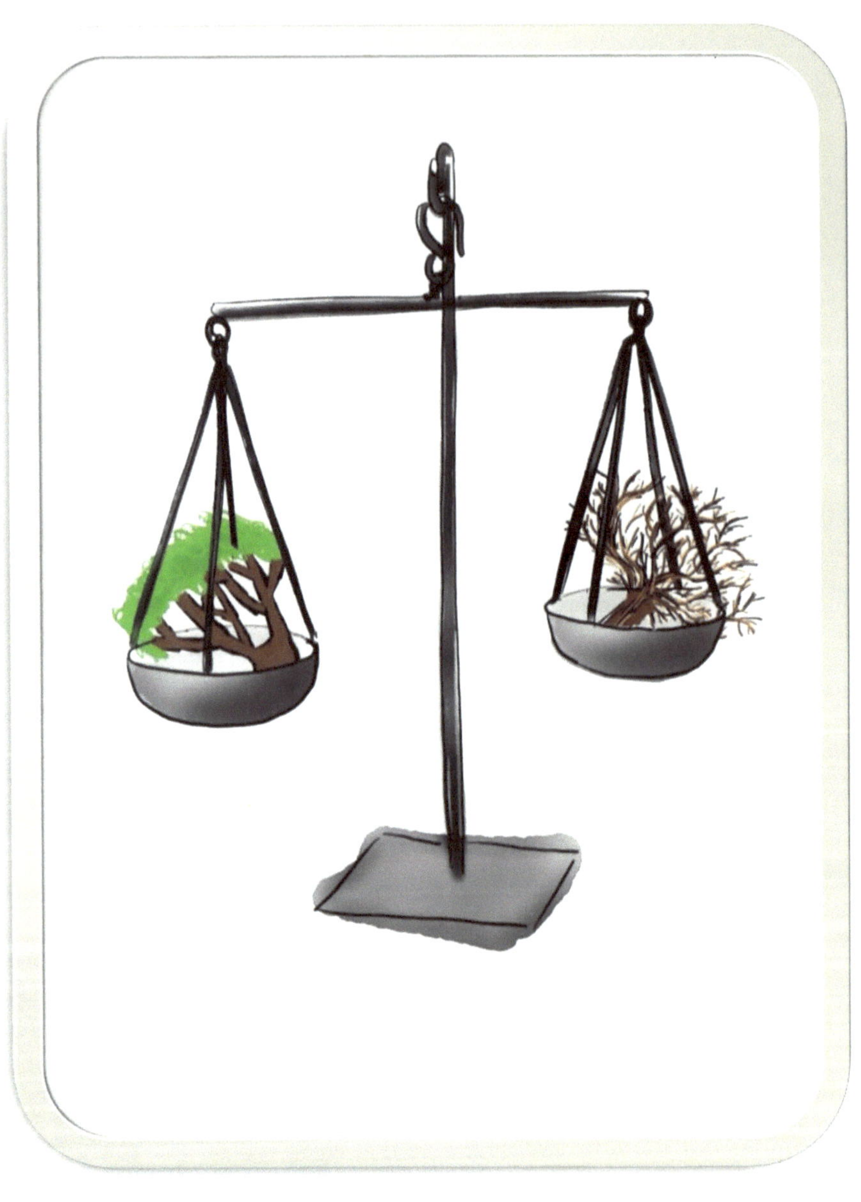

Polarity

By Misna Burelli

One of the most famous quotes attributed to Carl Jung is, "No tree… can grow to heaven unless its roots reach down to hell".[22] Many of us intuitively understand the essence of the quote, acknowledging its truth. Jordan Peterson also values this quote because it is profound, touching one of life's greatest mysteries: polarity.[23]

Polarity has been a recurring concept throughout history and many disciplines. From Taoism to great psychoanalysts such as Jung, societies and individuals have theorized about it. We all know about the yin and yang or the dark side versus the light as an often-observed element of polarity.

But what is polarity? One could reduce it to a simple plus versus minus on a scale where the middle is neutral. Or alternatively, a yes or no to a clear-cut question. But usually it is more complicated than that. Perhaps we should say polarity is something that expresses itself on opposite ends of a spectrum, where the root cause or the fundamental basic origin is the same.

Unsurprisingly, homeopathic remedies often contain components of polarity of varying degrees, generating additional confirmatory tools for archetype selection. This fairly new field of research was founded by the Swiss homeopath Heiner Frei and has been called "polarity analysis".[24] One of the advantages of polarity analysis is that certain remedies can be excluded based on contraindications. This clears the field so that the pool of remaining remedies becomes much smaller. It can also be adapted to computer analysis.

Keeping in mind that polarity can show on the physical, mental, and emotional levels, it could present itself like this on the physical plane:

---

[22] Jung, C.G. and the C.G. Jung Foundation for Analytical Psychology www.cgjungny.org

[23] Peterson, J.B. *12 Rules for Life: An Antidote to Chaos*, Random House Canada, **2018,** page 180

[24] Frei, H. Polarity analysis, a new approach to increase the precision of homeopathic prescriptions *Homeopathy* **2009,** *98*: 49-5

if a remedy picture has thirst as one of its main characteristics, the opposite is also often true, even though it might be less common. Therefore, either the archetype is really thirsty or completely thirstless, but not in between. This is only true when the archetype is off balance, of course. In the middle, between the two poles, the archetype would be feeling just right—not too thirsty and not too thirstless. That is the state we are aiming for when complete healing has taken place.

The above is an example of polarity displayed on the physical plane, but we can notice such things happening on all levels. Let's see how this could play out on the mental/emotional plane. Suppose a person named Jack is very healthy. Looking at him, one can observe mostly positive personality or character traits. But as his health weakens, he loses these positive attributes, and what was originally a strength, will now become a liability. It could appear like this:

Jack is detail oriented and works in an environment with numbers—a tax office. He is happy, as he has a natural ability to check and double check records; he is extremely reliable, consistently ensuring that things are 150% correct. His job is perfect for him because the environment fits his personality, and he is satisfied and successful.

But now imagine him sick. Where is he most vulnerable? There are two possibilities: he could become tired, losing concentration, performing poorly, mixing up numbers and forgetting what he wanted to do. Losing his edge. Letting his job become a monotonous drudgery at an uninspiring 50% effort. Or, on the flip side, he could over-do what he's good at. He could perform at 300% instead of 150%. So, you say that's even better? At first glance, it may appear advantageous. However, at that level of meticulousness, he's bogging down and stressing out over every new client, going home too late, and letting things move too slowly; he's too stubborn and never satisfied with the result. Others will inevitably start avoiding him because he's too detail oriented, becoming a difficult person to work with. They will notice that things get stuck in his office. Ultimately, his reputation will suffer. His greatest strength will become his greatest weakness as his health deteriorates.

This is just one example, but there are countless others because polarity is a principle. Polarities are the extreme tendencies we have when we are unwell. Every remedy picture has these polarities and when balanced and healthy they are mostly invisible—not too much and not too little of the peculiarities, strengths and weaknesses that make up the archetype. But when times are bad—when the equilibrium between the planes and the body as a whole is disturbed—even former strengths can become real liabilities, and former liabilities are not useful, without the context of the positive pole.

Another common case of polarities extending too far to one side often happens around compassion. Even though the healthy range of emotions can reach pretty far on both sides, there have recently been some very clear cases of people going overboard with their feelings in one direction only. In their overly positive state, these formerly great warriors for truth, justice, and equality, have now shifted their goal to help the unfortunate into a kind of self-abandoning tournament. In their attempt to stand out and save the world, their priorities get mixed up, and they cannot distinguish between worthy goals, realistic goals, and self-destructive goals. Their objective is now only compassion, no matter the price.

Anxiety and depression follow the same patterns. The target is not to aim for an anxiety level of zero on the far side of the positive pole. Anxiety is a useful warning signal that keeps you out of trouble when confronted with uncertainty and danger. But too much anxiety makes life miserable. It's like living with the alarm permanently set on emergency. And that would be life on the edge of the negative pole.

The same is true for depression. On the positive end of the pole we can't and shouldn't demand to only have blissfully happy days. To never feel unhappy would make us into robots. We should mourn our losses and feel our pains just like humans do, but we should not get so overwhelmed that we can't cope; we should not behave like someone just died every day, which is the end of the negative pole. The state with both emotions present is the most appropriate.

Let's go back to Jung's "tree quote" (no tree... can grow to heaven unless its roots reach down to hell) and see how it applies to this. The quote represents the ideal balanced archetype with strong characteristics covering both positive and negative poles. The unbalanced positive archetype would be too much of a good thing. With the negative pole missing, this could be a person that's way too innocent, nice, and trusting, eventually becoming a victim of bullying. The outcome will be self-destruction or enslavement, simply because there is no self-preservation. The unbalanced negative archetype would be this: not enough of a good thing which could lead all the way from being too difficult, suspicious, mean, aggressive, violent, without a conscience, to outright evil. Since there is nothing good left in this case, it's more obvious that it will lead straight to disaster.

Being on both pole ends is problematic, while the middle, which contains parts of both poles, is the ideal and strongest archetype. If you cannot identify the middle, where self-protection and compassion are both adequately present, you are vulnerable to both extremes, because as soon as you realize that one pole gave you dangerous exposure to being abused, you switch over to the other side, which is full of revenge and bitterness. The rage that can set in here puts you straight on the far negative end of the spectrum—into the "hell" area.

Sometimes I see commentary that's missing the point. People who say, "what nonsense, Jung's quote is encouraging me to be evil!". This is a complete misinterpretation and shows a lack of understanding reality as it is. It is not he, who has the *most evil* within, is also the strongest, nor he who is strongest must be evil. Instead, it is he who has both *some* evil and good parts *balanced together*, in the right way, will be strongest. It's the balance that counts!

The danger that pole extremes switch sides can happen in many ways. For example, when a workaholic is suddenly too exhausted to work, or violent revolutionaries give up and withdraw in frustration, they will internalize their feelings in an unhealthy, self-destructive way. Or again, when a bully becomes a coward, after being confronted by an even bigger bully. For individuals, societies, and the world as a whole, it is a good idea to stay in the middle. Weak, imbalanced archetypes, at the pole extremes, are much more dangerous than strong, balanced ones, even though the middle always contains parts of both extremes.

Even without thinking homeopathically, polarities give people a chance to foresee how they might be vulnerable, allowing them to take active steps to prevent sliding onto the pole extremes. If I know, for example, that I tend to be a workaholic, I might be very careful to watch myself. Maybe my work attitude has served me well in terms of career and success, but I can tell that sometimes I have the tendency to go overboard with it. This tendency of "too much of a good thing" might wreck my health and push me off balance. Therefore, I might be on the lookout for burnout, the other side of the spectrum. I might make it a point to accept related criticism from my husband or wife without reacting angrily. I might also try to analyze the situation and find out why I'm off balance—be it a stressful work situation or a health problem. If you want to know more about this, you can look up your homeopathic archetype and check out how it looks like when it is sick. This will give you insight into your vulnerabilities.

It is true that we, as humans, have trouble coping with the concept of polarity. It makes us uneasy to find both poles within us, and some of us think that seeing the "shadow"—as Jung calls the other side—is pathological and should be avoided at all cost. It can feel good, out there on the pole ends, because without doubting that we are doing the right thing, we feel morally superior. Ignorance is bliss. But that is not what we want. We want to incorporate the shadow in a productive and balanced manner. We should be strong enough to deal with the shadow. We should work on it. Similarly, if we understand Peterson's concept of consciousness and meaning as the middle between order and chaos, we recognize that he is saying the same thing. His recommendation to "position yourself where the terror of existence is under control and you are secure, but where you are also alert and engaged" is meant as advice to place yourself between the positive and negative pole—into the productive and life affirming section of the spectrum. He is making a case *against* extreme polarity and *for* balance.[25]

To sum it up: Polarity is a universal principle that is visible everywhere in our society (or in the universe?) that affects everyone—

---

[25] Peterson, J.B. *12 Rules for Life: An Antidote to Chaos*, Random House Canada, **2018**, pages 35-44

including you! It is obvious that we, as a society, have become more unbalanced recently. Many people have become so polarized that they can't even talk to others from the opposing camp. That is what it means to be polarized: to not have even a little bit of the other side inside you and to not understand the other side at all. It is clearly a dangerous path we are on. An imbalanced path. Just like the archetype who needs both opposing poles, our society needs to be able to accommodate these opposite viewpoints without hate, blame and major unrest. If we are not able to do that peacefully and find our true middle, extreme polarity will take us over the edge and it doesn't even matter which side of the cliff we fall off because usually the two opposing ends are connected more than we would like to admit and can easily morph into each other. They are two sides of the same coin.

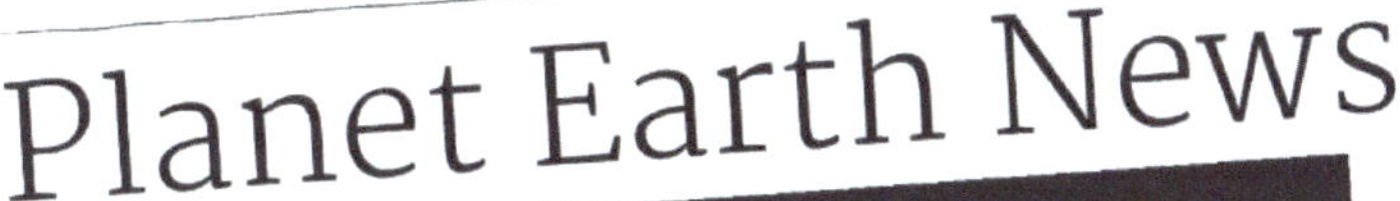

Interview with Carl Jung: His Explanation of "The Shadow"

The Devouring Mother: Carl Jung called me a Gorgon exclusive details on page 5

****

In his own words: Hahnemann stole my research!

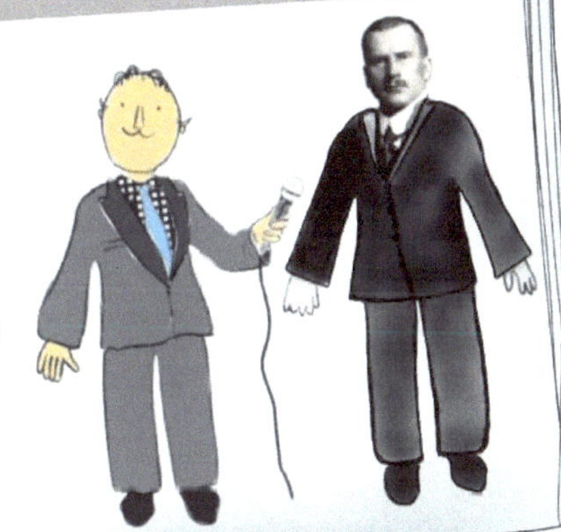

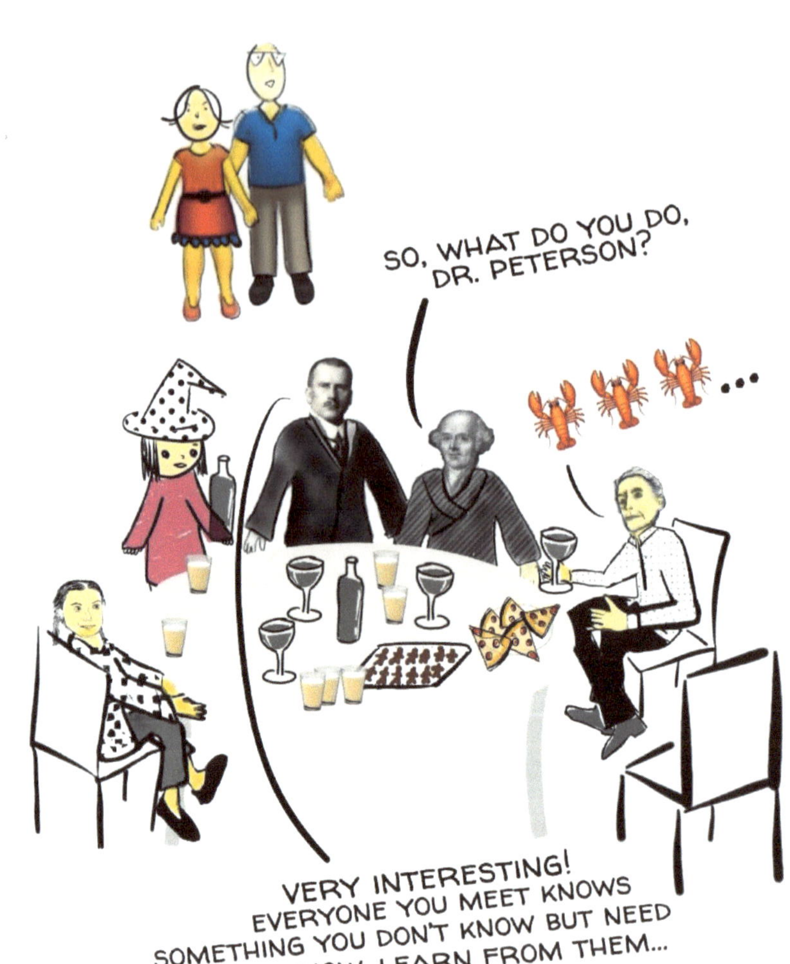
SO, WHAT DO YOU DO, DR. PETERSON?
...
VERY INTERESTING!
EVERYONE YOU MEET KNOWS
SOMETHING YOU DON'T KNOW BUT NEED
TO KNOW...LEARN FROM THEM...

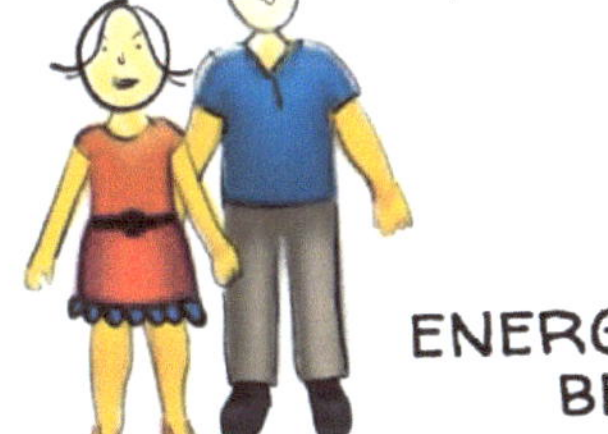

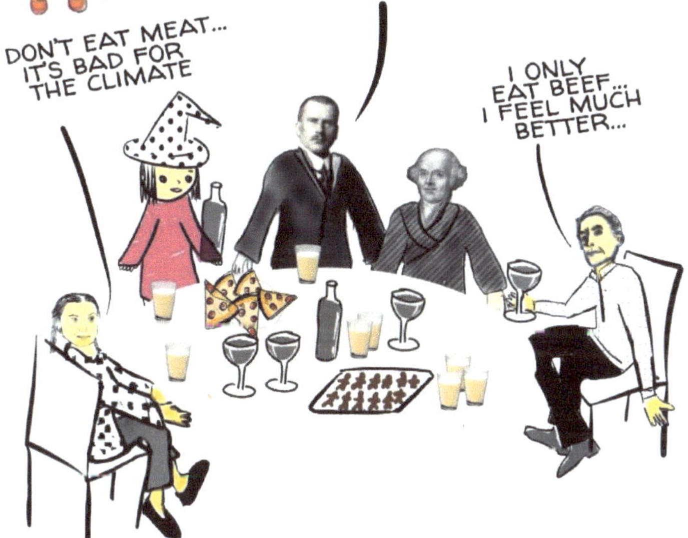
ENERGY ITSELF IS A TENSION BETWEEN OPPOSITES
I DON'T EAT MEAT... IT'S BAD FOR THE CLIMATE
I ONLY EAT BEEF... I FEEL MUCH BETTER...

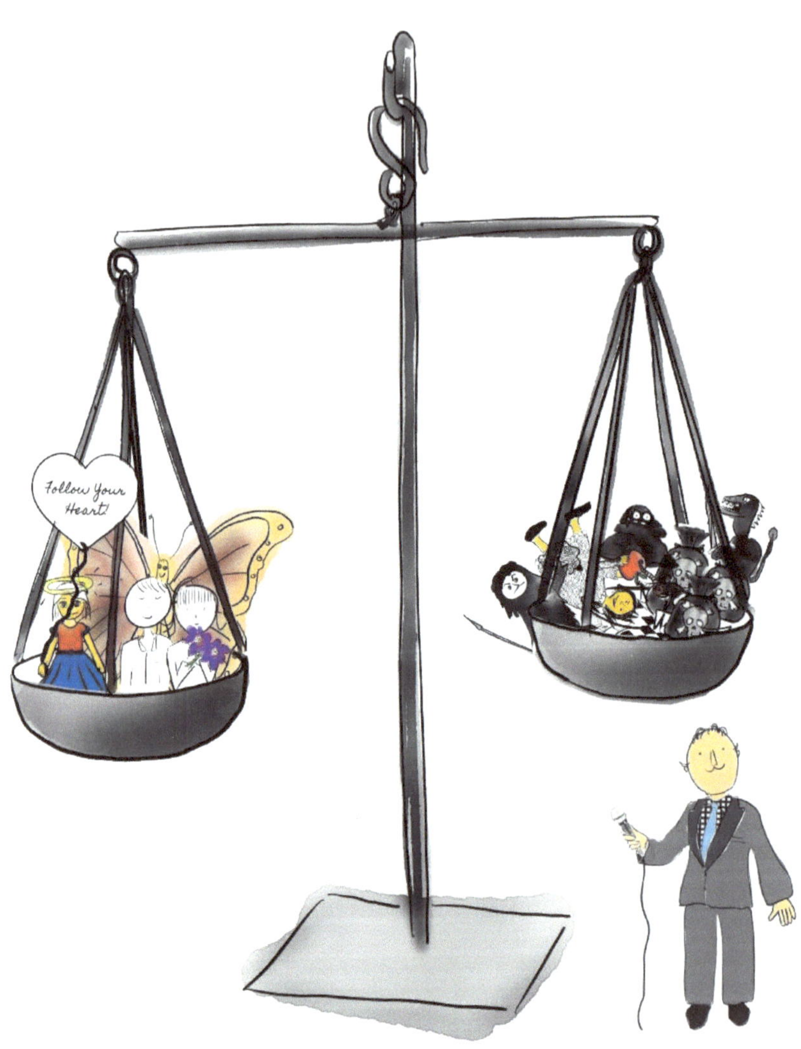
Follow Your
Heart!

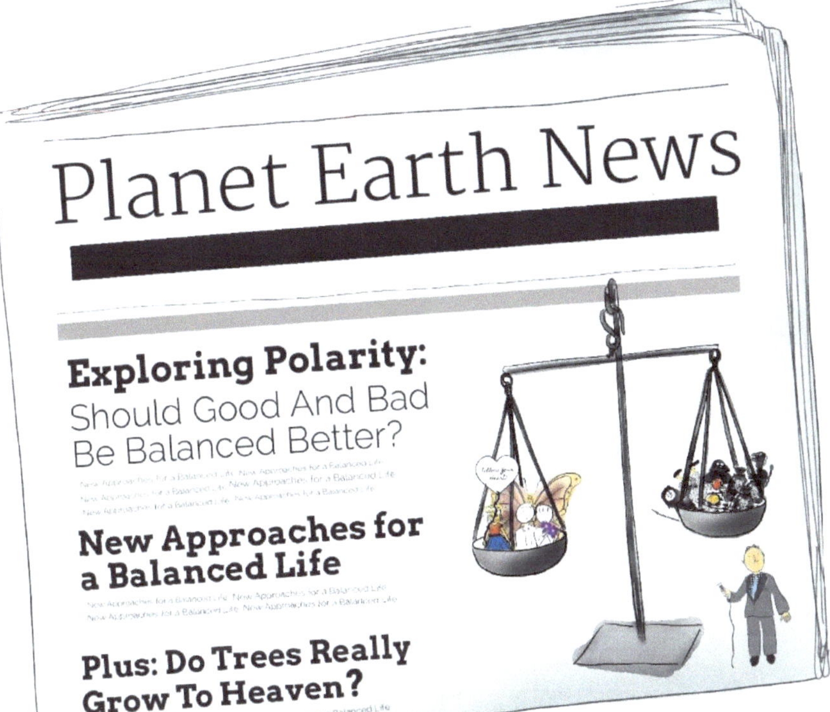
Planet Earth News
Exploring Polarity:
Should Good And Bad
Be Balanced Better?
New Approaches for
a Balanced Life
Plus: Do Trees Really
Grow To Heaven?

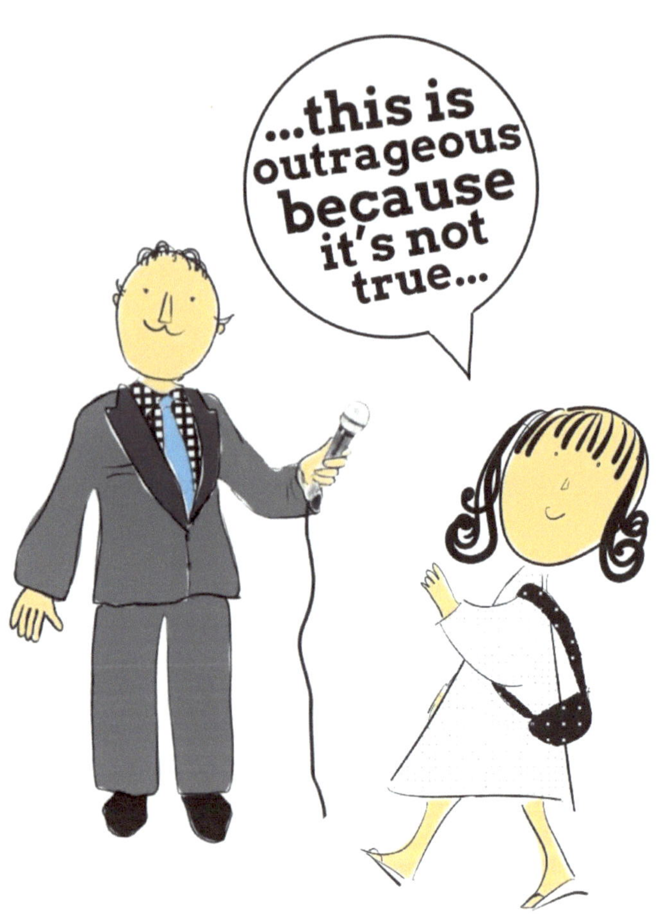
...this is outrageous because it's not true...

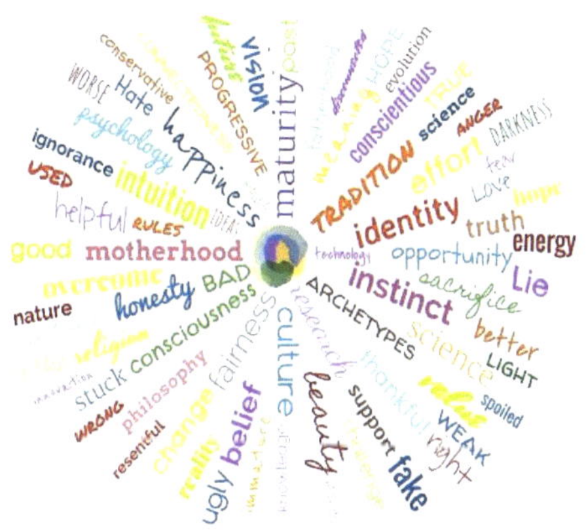
conservative
WORSE
Hate
psychology
ignorance
USED
intuition
helpful
RULES
happiness
PROGRESSIVE
VISION
maturity
past
evolution
conscientious
science
ANGER
DARKNESS
TRADITION
effort
Love
hope
identity
truth
energy
good
motherhood
technology
opportunity
nature
honesty
BAD
instinct
sacrifice
Lie
consciousness
ARCHETYPES
science
better
LIGHT
stuck
religion
fairness
culture
research
philosophy
WRONG
resentful
change
belief
reality
ugly
beauty
support
thankful
value
spoiled
WEAK
right
fake

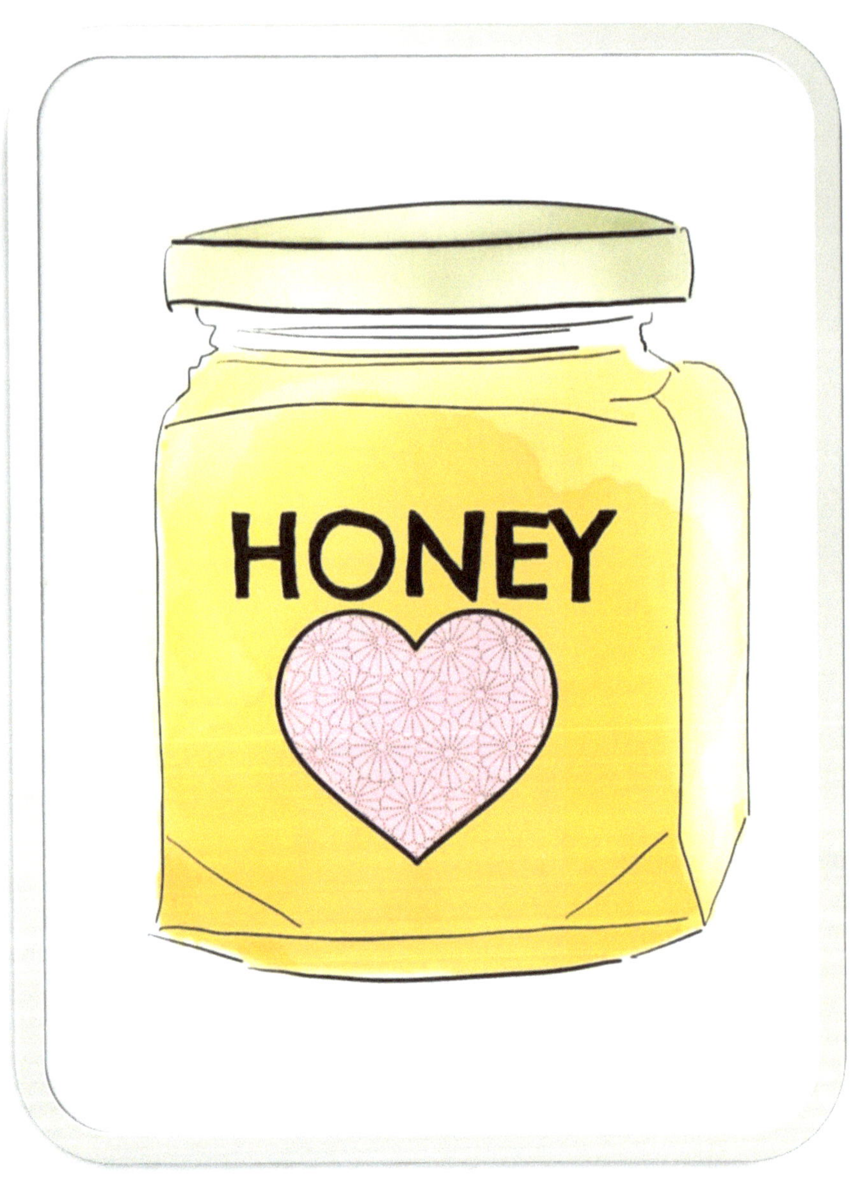
HONEY

Archetype Perceptions

By Lena Kratz

Today, there are thousands of different homeopathic remedies, each with their own archetype picture. However, most cases only require remedies from the most common archetypes. These common remedies are called polychrests, and there are about twenty of them. Their archetypes are well-known and have been solid for a couple of centuries.

In addition, it turns out that many common substances have widespread archetype perceptions in the population. Here is a list:

For example, *saccharum officinale* (sugar), as a remedy, is associated with archetype themes of love, self-love, and unfulfilled love, and we, as a culture, seem to know it, calling each other honey or sweetie, and singing "sugar pie, honey bun". Another example might be *silica* (sand, glass) which is known to "need grit", as in "needs to be more courageous". It "breaks but will not bend", just like the silica personality, which is stubborn. *Ferrum metallicum* (iron) is well-known for its "iron will and iron fist", a striking emotional symptom of the archetype. *Cuprum metallicum* (copper) has a pretty similar emotional archetype to what we think a "cop"(per)—a police man—should be like, illustrating this concept perfectly. The *aurum metallicum* (gold) archetype "shines", but is "heavy with responsibility", and tends to take things very seriously ("heavy and quiet"). It expects a gold medal performance from itself and is extremely driven. Unsurprisingly, it is found among the most successful, the highest achievers. But if things don't work out as expected, a disappointed "heaviness" can set in, pushing the individual off track, leading to major depression—*did someone say polarity?*

Of all these metals, *argentum metallicum* (silver) conducts electricity and heat the best, preventing the *argentum metallicum* archetype from retaining its body heat, resulting in always feeling cold—it can't keep its temperature on the physical plane. On the emotional plane this archetype tends to be anxious, creative and a good public speaker "silver-tongued", "speech is silver—silence is gold". *Platinum metallicum* (platinum) is similarly driven as the gold archetype—*platinum metallicum* individuals are often very successful—but suffers from arrogance, keeping a distance to "lesser" individuals while believing they are "better".

A really intriguing example of archetype perception is the picture of *lycopodium clavatum*, a remedy made from running pine, which is a plant in the family of club mosses or ground pines. The plant looks like small pine trees. Once upon a time, these "ground pines" used to be fairly large trees, but today, they are only small mosses, usually seen growing in wooded areas. Interestingly, it seems as if the plant has not managed to get over its loss of stature, as the main emotional characteristic of the archetype is low self-esteem, along with a correlated desire to brag, cheat, and make oneself look bigger than one actually is. The remedy is associated both with bullying and servitude, and there is often a distinct desire to please higher authorities. We can see the polarity—intimidation and victimization occur at the same time but the reason for the behavior is rooted in low self-esteem.

There are more such correlations, but I picked some of these well-known and interesting examples to explain the concept. In these cases, people's perceptions of a substance manage to nail the mental/emotional archetype associated with the remedy.

On a more professional level, a branch of homeopathy founded by Rajan Sankaran, called the sensation method, is based on these kinds of perceptions of natural substances as archetype pictures—you find the correct remedy by recognizing the natural substance in yourself.[26] This approach has been a relatively recent addition to the homeopathic method but has been growing in popularity over the last few years.

Perceptions of natural substances and associated archetypes play a large role in everyday life and how we judge others. Movies are full of them. Analyzing movie characters according to archetypes can be fun because—as Jung and von Franz have pointed out—these archetypes are known by intuition.[27] We humans can all recognize tried and true

---

[26] Sankaran, R. *The Other Song: Discovering Your Parallel Self*, Homeopathic Medical Publishers, **2008**

[27] Von Franz, M. *Archetypal Dimensions of the Psyche*, Shambhala Boston & London, **1997,** p.6

characters appearing throughout history, such as characters from the bible, for example, if they follow, "mythical primal ideas, which take a similar form in all human beings".[22] Movies and books are a lot better when the characters come across as authentic, fitting some known typical picture—something that people have seen before in real life—resonating with them because the story touches the truth. "Real" personalities can be weak or strong, showing their coping skills; unavoidable hardships present challenges we long to follow, catching a glimpse of their lives—but this is only interesting if the characters are genuine. Good movie directors and actors know these secrets and pay attention to the authenticity of the script. When they don't follow these unwritten rules, characters often appear artificial and the movie flops.

Have you seen good movie archetypes like that? You probably have, intuitively recognizing this fact. Take Harry Potter,[28] from the *Harry Potter* book series, for example. Why is he such a convincing example of a true hero? He is courageous, smart, and resilient, with just the right amount of moral fiber, and he also has a small fragment of evil embedded within himself which he is able to handle very well. Being a strong character, he needs some aspects of polarity, but the negative pole doesn't define him. Instead, it gives him the opportunity to truly understand what the other side is capable of, helping him defeat it. Of course, there is danger associated with this, making the story more exhilarating.

How about a totally different character—Anakin Skywalker, aka Darth Vader from *Star Wars*. In contrast to Harry, Anakin is weak, initially a nice and innocent boy who fears abandonment and losing people dear to him. In an attempt to avoid pain and suffering, a number of bad, impulsive decisions, produce the exact situation that he's so afraid of, hurting him where he is most vulnerable. Anakin has no principles, is easily hurt, feels treated unfairly, and follows just about anyone.

Anakin then demonstrates his weakness when he flips to the

---

[28] Rowling, J.K. *Harry Potter* (books 1-7), Arthur A. Levine Books, Box edition **2007**

"dark side", turning into the angry and vengeful Darth Vader. But even the all-powerful Darth Vader is still a weak character who becomes a tool of the emperor, following the emperor's every command.

These familiar circumstances confirm again that there is more danger and disorganization out on the pole extremes than in the middle.

Both Darth Vader and Harry Potter, weak and strong as they are, resonate with us because they follow known archetype pictures. They seem to be cut from the fabric of human drama that we see all around us and thus appear believable.

And even though learning to recognize and analyze archetypes in depth could be a useful skill in the business world or around social relationships, this is not a concept that is usually taught in schools. It requires a kind of "stepping out of oneself" and being able to take an honest look back at what one is doing. Obviously, this can be awkward at first. Some people describe this process as mindfulness, a way of thinking about oneself and one's place in the world. Even though we don't often come across mindfulness being taught in schools and colleges, there are some exceptions, such as Joshua Spodek's entrepreneurship classes, and his book, *Leadership Step by Step*.[29] I really like his book because it teaches self-awareness, not just by way of theory, but through actual practice exercises. Analyzing archetypes is much easier from a higher level of self-awareness—the goal of this book.

There are some interesting quotes by Jung that touch this subject exactly. As Jung famously said, "everything that irritates us about others can lead us to an understanding of ourselves... [and] until you make the unconscious conscious it will direct your life, and you will call it fate". In our modern-day polarized states, we are not only less tolerant of other points of view, but overall more fragile as individuals. Covering up our feelings of discomfort, rather than confronting them, we abuse alcohol or other substances. To become aware, responsible and tolerant, we would have to explore both poles, something we are unwilling or unable to do in our damaged states. Emerging consciousness can set in motion

---

[29] Spodek, J. *Leadership Step by Step: become the person others follow* Amacom Books, New York, **2017**

a painful process, accompanied by deep disappointments, even loss of friendships, but, as Jung would undoubtedly tell you, it is well worth the effort. Even though avoiding reality is endemic in current culture, it cannot be a long-term solution.

Fortunately, things will often fall into place for those of us who are open to it—as we work on reaching a higher level of health this will happen automatically. We will cover some of these topics in later chapters.

But back to the remedy archetypes. At this point people usually inquire about all the remedies they have seen at local stores, highlighting the obvious inconsistency that none of the bottles list archetypes—no personality traits are involved in purchasing a remedy! That is true because in those cases the remedies are meant to be used for acute conditions only, with the bottles listing a short summary of symptoms to be treated. This really only works for emergencies, and for a very limited time, while people are the "injured archetype" or the "high dry fever archetype" or the "ear ache in cranky babies while teething archetype". Even though all these conditions come with emotional—and sometimes even mental symptoms—as well, such details are too short lived, and are typically ignored when remedies are sold at local pharmacies or grocery stores. We could call such states simply temporary archetypes. And if the physical picture, such as an injury, is very clear, the remedy works just fine without the complicated and distracting mental/emotional picture.

There is a whole branch of homeopathy dedicated to finding ways for easier remedy matching by using a clear medical diagnosis, such as a urinary tract infection or high blood cholesterol, as a basis for up to three remedy suggestions. The initial research for this approach has come from the Banerji Family of doctors in India,[30] who have used it for many decades, but recently it has been brought into the US by Joette Calabrese,[31] who has studied extensively with the Banerjis. It is an interesting method that could simplify remedy selection by avoiding the

---

[30] Banerji, B. and Banerji, P. *The Banerji Protocols: A New Method of Treatment with Homeopathic Medicines*, Pratip Banerji, Kolkata, India, **2013**

[31] Calabrese, J. at Joettecalabrese.com

challenging constitutional picture.

Although applicable to certain chronic diseases, this type of diagnoses-based remedy selection is somewhat limited in its scope because today we are often dealing with complicated long-term chronic conditions, developmental delays in children or uncleared miasms.

As will become clear in the next chapter, acute and chronic diseases are linked: it's hard to cure one when you suppress the other. Perhaps this is the time to take a look at these relationships.

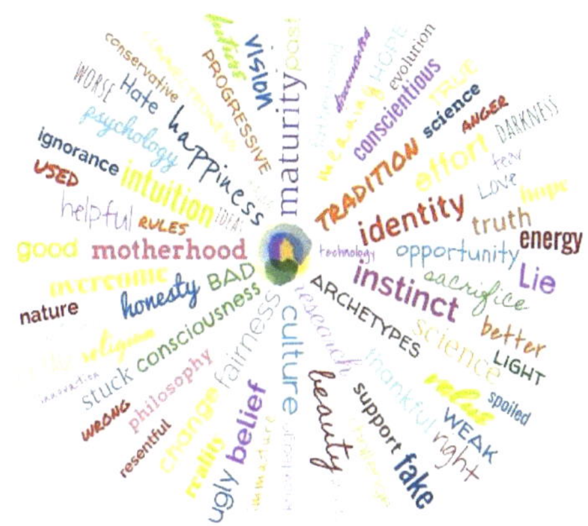
conservative
WORSE
Hate
psychology
happiness
PROGRESSIVE
VISION
maturity
HOPE
evolution
conscientious
science
ANGER
DARKNESS
TRADITION
effort
LOVE
ignorance
USED
intuition
helpful
RULES
identity
truth
energy
good
motherhood
technology
opportunity
honesty
BAD
instinct
sacrifice
Lie
nature
consciousness
ARCHETYPES
better
stuck
philosophy
fairness
culture
science
LIGHT
WRONG
thankful
spoiled
resentful
change
beauty
support
WEAK
right
ugly
belief
fake

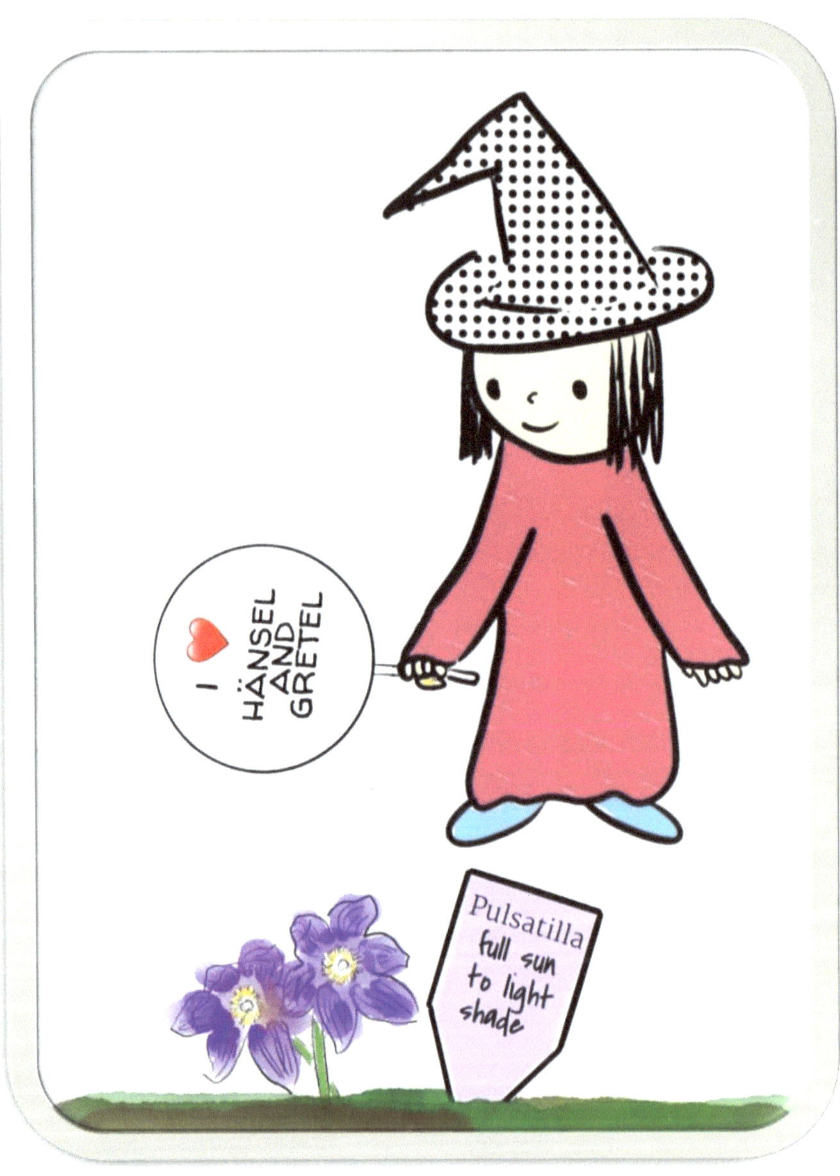
I ♥ HÄNSEL AND GRETEL
Pulsatilla
full sun to light shade

The Devouring Mother Archetype

By Lena Kratz

Let's talk about acute diseases versus chronic diseases: mental/emotional symptoms are typically more obvious in the latter—archetype pictures play a much larger role there, with the mental/emotional state potentially even replacing the physical picture.

Looking at the case of a simple strep throat (streptococcus pyogenes), noting that empty swallowing hurts a lot while swallowing solid food feels better, and that the tonsils are sprinkled with creamy white dots and look bright red, we could probably find a suitable remedy in a store. Throw in a high or low fever, a fast or slow onset, and we should be assured of success.

But what if the strep throat becomes chronic? The sore throat might morph into a condition called PANDAS (Pediatric Autoimmune Neuropsychiatric Disorders Associated with Streptococcal Infections).[32] PANDAS consists almost exclusively of long-term mental/emotional symptoms, being described as a mixture of severe anxiety, OCD, tics, and aggression, often rendering school children unable to attend classes. The painfully red throat might not be visible at all, preventing us from finding a remedy. No matter what, we would not choose to address this syndrome with emergency remedies: the full archetypal picture needs to be evaluated under those circumstances.

The strep infection that is responsible for the problematic behavioral symptoms extends deeper onto the mental/emotional plane than it should—it is not supposed to reach there! But nowadays, in many cases, it does, and homeopathy can explain why it happens: suppression.

There are a number of typical childhood remedies needed by almost every child at one point or another, treating acute conditions such as fevers, coughs, the flu, or a stomach bug, but also the particular state that the child is in. Rather than being constitutional remedies, these are

[32] Maloney, B.A. *Saving Sammy, a mothers fight to cure her son's OCD* Three Rivers Press, New York **2009**

just common transient archetype states, which will be resolved on the way to adulthood. You could treat them as temporary archetypes or let the child go through the state naturally; both are appropriate. But these days, standard procedure demands that we suppress the illness with fever reducing (or other) medications, eliminating painful symptoms to the point of not even looking sick any longer.

Have you noticed that when children are acutely ill, they often make a huge developmental jump after the illness passes? We saw it once in our daughter—she suddenly seemed to be so much more mature! Coincidence? Perhaps not! It has been noted in older literature and used to be something that people actually paid attention to in the olden days. Nowadays, no one even notices it—probably because it doesn't exist anymore! With all the symptom suppressing medication being thrown at children, they are no longer actually going through a natural case of infectious disease—and that may be a problem!

It turns out that plenty of mainstream conventional medical literature recognizes the link between the suppression of symptoms and the generation of a whole new set of diseases. One prime example of this phenomenon is the atopic march,[33] a condition that links children's eczema turning into asthma—after using suppressive cortisone cream on the itchy spots. This connection has been known for a long time, although doctors usually brush it off as coincidence.

Homeopaths teach this simple rule: suppressing the body's symptoms will push them deeper, causing them to become more serious long-term, both for acute and chronic conditions. Contrast this with allowing the body to produce symptoms: you might benefit, both from the developmental jump after the illness passes and from long-term health-protective mechanisms inherent in acute illness.[34] Is the fact that we are largely missing out on these processes the reason why we see so much chronic illness and immaturity everywhere? It would be worth exploring!

---

[33] Spergel, J.M. From atopic dermatitis to asthma: the atopic march *Ann. Allergy Asthma Immunol.* **2010**, *105(2)*:99-106

[34] Hoption Cann, S.A. et al. Acute infections as a means of cancer prevention: Opposing effects to chronic infections? *Cancer Detect. Prev.* **2006**, *30(1)*: 83-93

Let's take measles as an example. Acute cases of measles are often successfully treated with *pulsatilla*, a common remedy made from a flower. *Pulsatilla* usually improves the physical symptoms of measles—the physical plane—but does the emotional plane hold any significance? After all, there is a whole archetype picture associated with the remedy, including mental and emotional states. It might be worth exploring how *pulsatilla* expresses itself on the mental/emotional plane. Similarly, to how measles is called a "childhood disease" *pulsatilla* is often referred to as a "children's remedy", dealing with feelings of abandonment, often expressed as whining and attention getting. *Pulsatilla* children are clingy and cry easily, but they are generally good natured in their dependence—exactly what we expect from a small child.

In adults it is a different story: too much dependence in adulthood is ugly. The *pulsatilla* adult is often nice but manipulative, wanting to be taken care of and fearing abandonment; there is frequently a kind of childishness and immaturity. *Pulsatilla* archetypes are usually better from consolation, experience "April weather" emotions and a tendency toward being easily depressed, crying a lot, and feeling better for it—older literature often describes this state as feeling "forsaken". *Pulsatilla* adults often suffer from a type of naiveté that leads the archetype to trust and follow the wrong crowd without realizing it. In their needy state, their susceptibility to such peer pressure can lead them to participate in questionable activities, from inappropriate partying all the way to drug addiction.

Pulsatilla is often too nice: this works in a positive environment, when family is close by and people trust one another. Happy *pulsatilla* moms love to take care of their children at home, creating a family sanctuary; but they may also focus so much on their family that their children (and others) can't have a life. Predictably, they suffer when the children grow up and leave the house, precipitating a midlife crisis; in an effort to stay relevant, they keep meddling in their children's affairs. They are oversensitive and easily offended. Without family or friends, the *pulsatilla* archetype feels lost and abandoned. Depressed and lonely in college, immature young *pulsatilla* students don't know what to do with life. On the truly pathological end of the spectrum, things tend to get difficult, reflecting the immaturity and dependence in the remedy by becoming clingy and manipulative—they demand that others devote their lives to them. Do you see the polarity? Much too nice when depending on others, versus frustration, sadness, and anger, as soon as relationships are threatened, and feelings of abandonment arise. *Pulsatilla* is mostly a women's state, perhaps because men's immune systems are different? No matter what, society allows it to happen—our culture typically doesn't afford the same tolerance towards obviously clingy and immature men.

But back to *pulsatilla* as a children's remedy: being frequently used to cure childhood ailments, a childish immaturity and dependency are part of every level in the archetype—making it necessary to clear out the state before adulthood.

So, what is the connection to our previous discussion about measles? Because *pulsatilla* can be enormously helpful when dealing with a case of measles, we could speculate that whatever the disease is might be kind of an equivalent to the remedy. It follows that going through measles naturally might be akin to giving you a good dose of *pulsatilla*. For the longest time, this has happened to every child on this planet—does it clear out their immature state of childhood *pulsatilla*?

Going through measles naturally, and feeling the "developmental jump" after the illness, may mean that from now on you would have been: less childish, dependent, whiny, manipulative, moody and emotional, oversensitive, depressed, and more ready to take care of yourself, not feeling abandoned, able to make better decisions in life, less susceptible to drug addiction, and on your way to becoming a productive mature adult—not a bad outcome!

It looks like I am picking measles and the corresponding remedy arbitrarily from a number of well-known disease-remedy combinations, but to me, the measles are an especially interesting case—there is a lot of conventional research revolving around them, and *pulsatilla*, their main remedy, has been a rock solid archetype for a couple of centuries.

So, what is it that makes the measles so special? This: research, showing that getting naturally infected with the measles virus might protect [35] against cancer [36] and other [37] future chronic diseases.[38] But it became really interesting after watching a couple of Jordan Peterson's [39] YouTube videos on the Devouring Mother archetype—must-watch material for anyone interested in archetype theories of any kind. It is especially interesting to see well researched archetypal pictures being used in other disciplines, and it seems that his analysis resonates with a lot of people. Why? Could it be because the Devouring Mother archetype is a common pathology these days? We have seen and heard stories of parents—mostly mothers—who are helping to choose their college kid's cafeteria lunch. They call professors, explaining why their children should get special treatment, they write emails to their kid's classmates or soccer coaches, guiding their every step. Employers already know that some moms will inquire about their offspring's prospects of employment before their interviews.

This may seem a bit extreme, but most of us have gotten used to seeing the Devouring Mother pathology in action—on college campuses, in the workplace and in every neighborhood. Radio discussions about helicopter versus snowplow parents indicate that there is a problem. It is not even uncommon—and I am pretty sure that much of the pathology of the Devouring Mother archetype overlaps *a lot* with the female adult archetype of *pulsatilla*. In other words, to put it bluntly: does the well-known Devouring Mother archetype have a biological basis in the suppression of measles?

---

[35] Bluming, A.Z. et al. Regression of Burkitt's lymphoma in association with measles infection *Lancet,* **1971**, *2(7715)*: 105-6

[36] Zygiert, Z. Hodgkin's disease: remissions after measles *Lancet* **1971**, *1(7699)*:593

[37] Cowan, T. *Vaccines, Autoimmunity, and the Changing Nature of Childhood Illness*, Chapter 10, Chelsea Green Publishing, **2018**

[38] Kubota, Y. et al. Association of measles and mumps with cardiovascular disease: The Japan Collaborative Cohort (JACC) study *Atherosclerosis* **2015,** *241(2)*:682-6

[39] Jordanbpeterson.com and Peterson, J.B. *12 Rules for Life: An Antidote to Chaos*, Random House Canada, **2018**

Planet Earth News

Interview with Al Ehrgy:
Smart, Honest And Always Concerned About His Students

Tragic friendships with pathogens: when we don't want to be healthy

General Fairfite and the golden rule: brings balance to life, avoids polarization BUT: don't forget to respect yourself! details on page 10

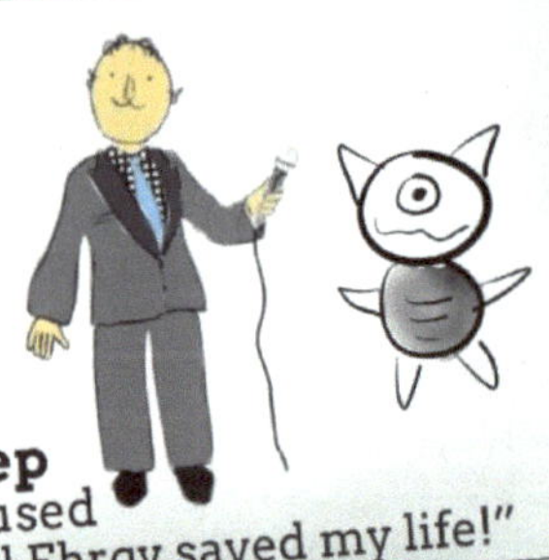

When you feel sorry for Strep: one recruit's personal story about his friendship with Strep bacteria "it felt good...I was confused and then it was almost too late... Al Ehrgy saved my life!"

Peace through Strength
Golden Rules
Integrity
do the right thing
Balance

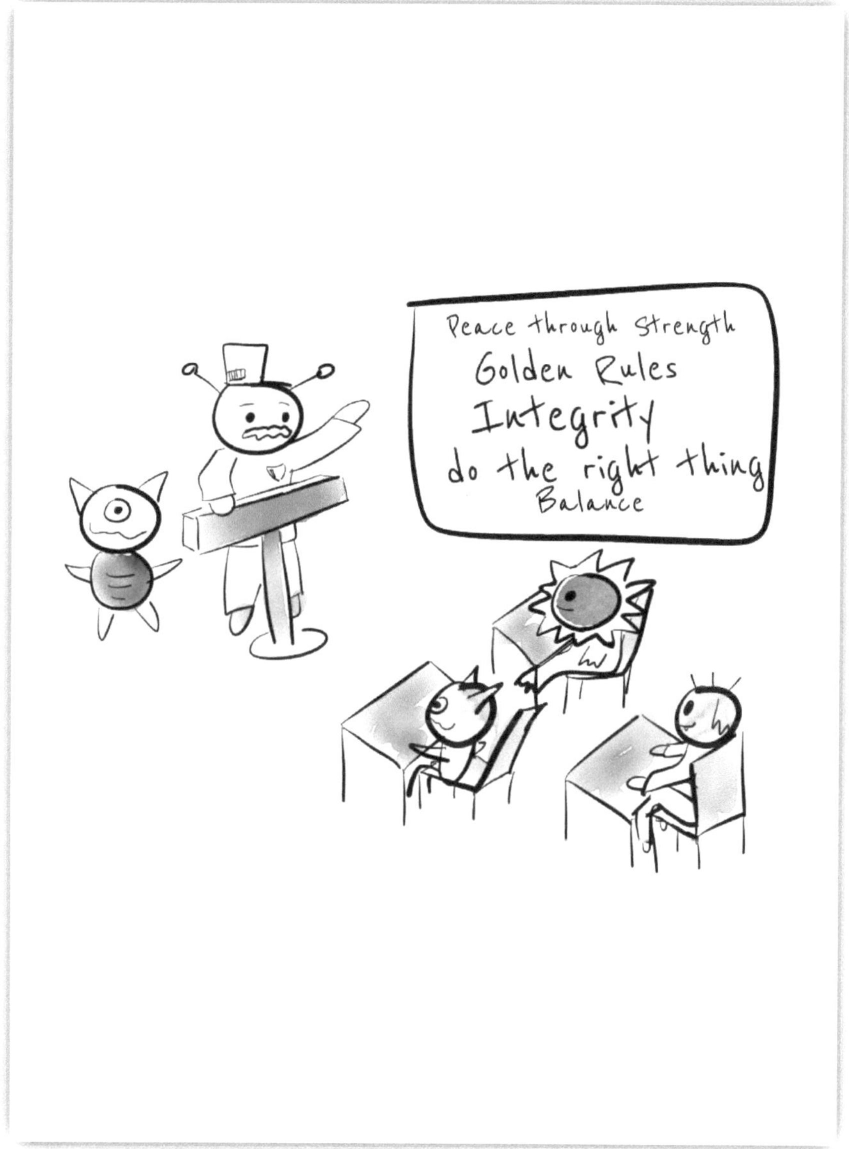

Immune System Lecture Notes

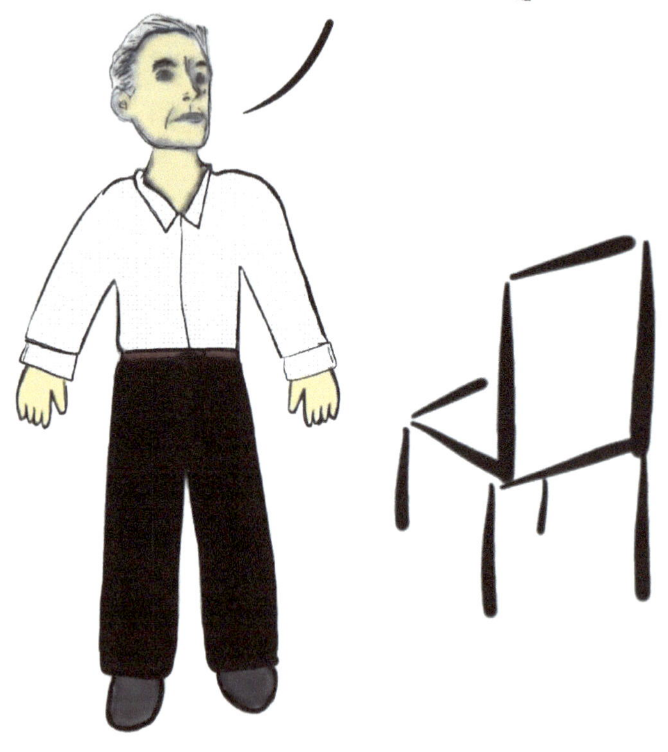
WHEN YOU HAVE SOMETHING TO SAY, SILENCE IS A LIE

THIS IS TOO GOOD TO BE TRUE...
I PLANTED IT... IT'S A PULSATILLA FLOWER!
WHAT A PRETTY FLOWER!
SURE, I AM FEEDING THEM... BUT I AM ALSO FEEDING OFF OF THEM...

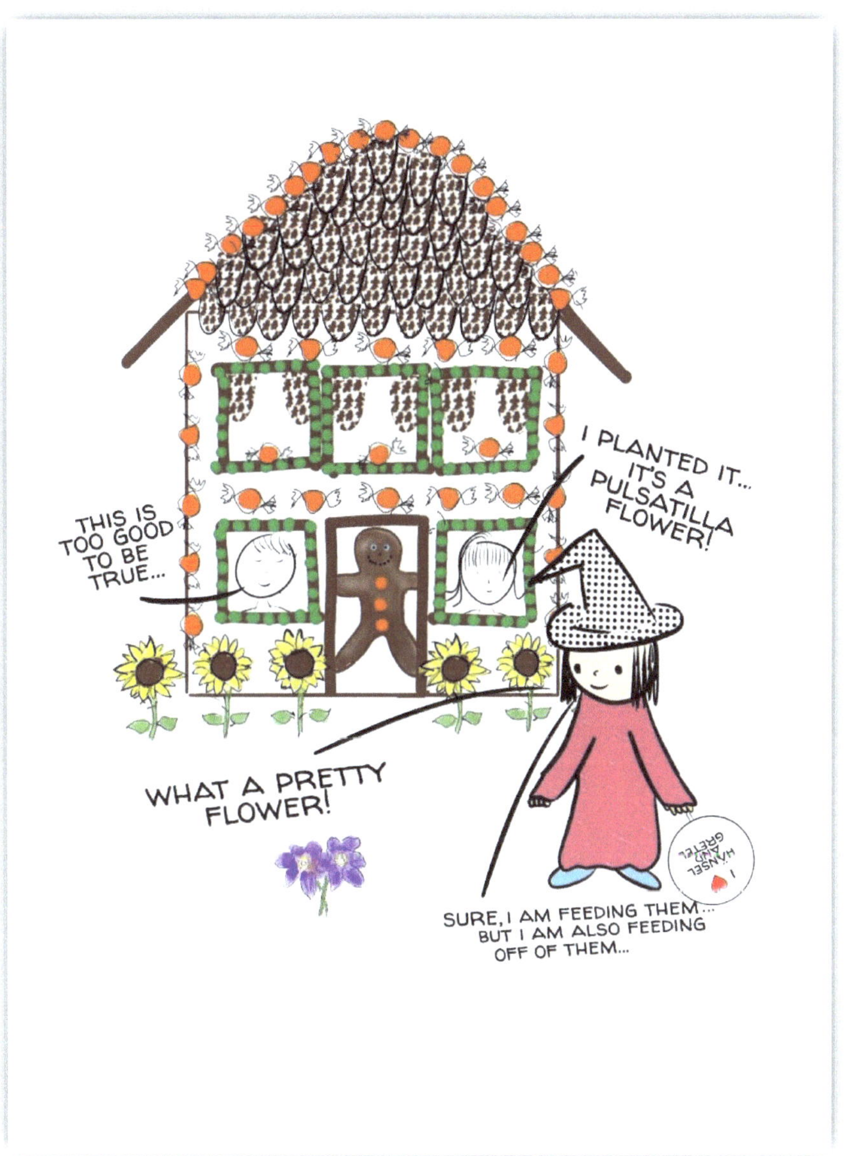

Homeopathic Fairy Tales:
Hänsel and Gretel

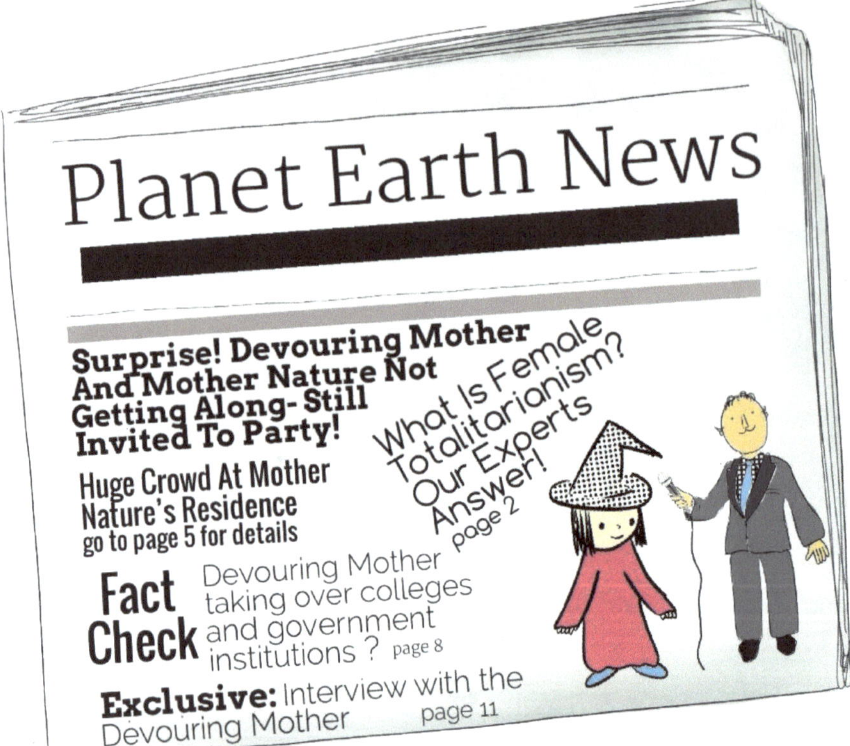

Planet Earth News

Surprise! Devouring Mother And Mother Nature Not Getting Along- Still Invited To Party!

Huge Crowd At Mother Nature's Residence
go to page 5 for details

What Is Female Totalitarianism? Our Experts Answer!
page 2

Fact Check
Devouring Mother taking over colleges and government institutions ? page 8

Exclusive: Interview with the Devouring Mother page 11

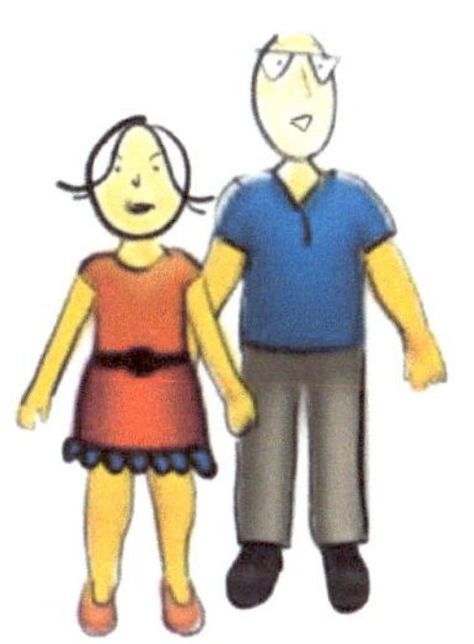

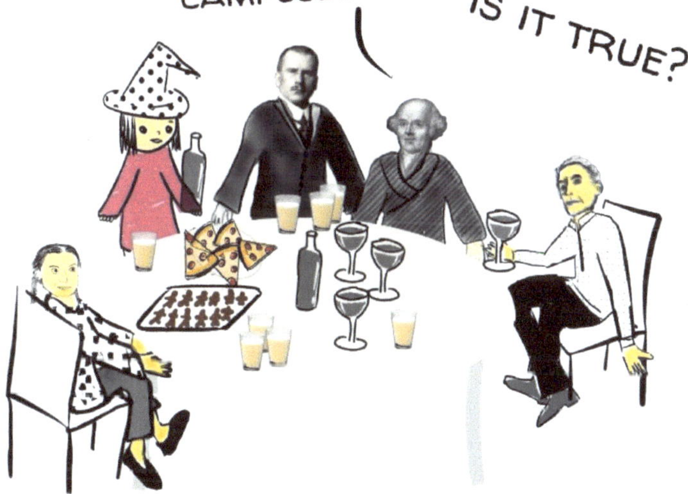
SO...DEVOURING MOTHER...
I HEARD THAT YOU ARE
TAKING OVER COLLEGE
CAMPUSES...
IS IT TRUE?

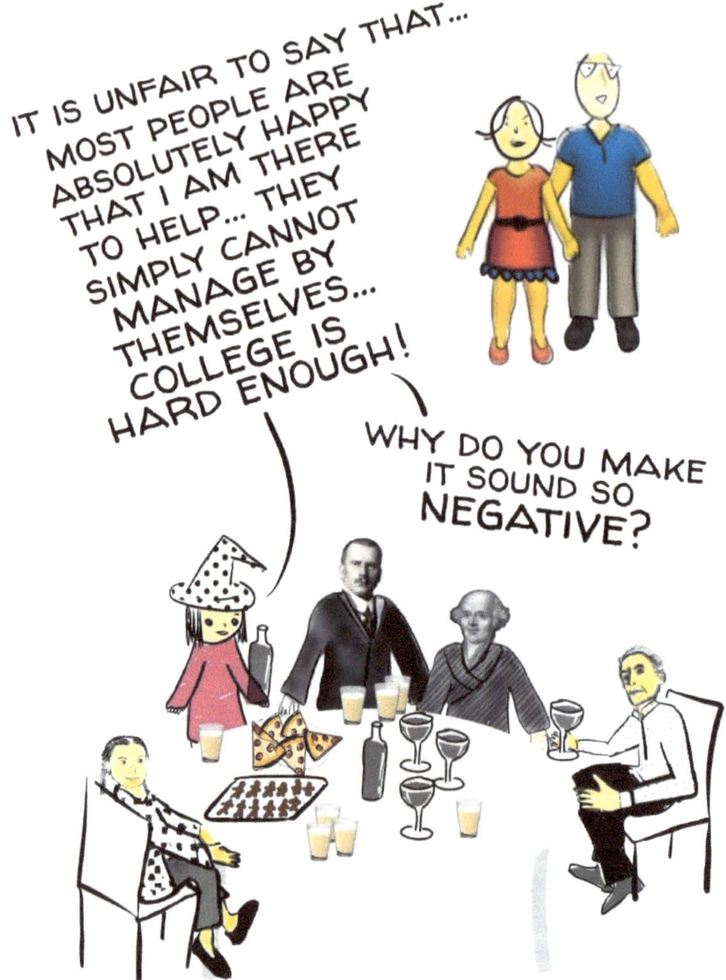
IT IS UNFAIR TO SAY THAT... MOST PEOPLE ARE ABSOLUTELY HAPPY THAT I AM THERE TO HELP... THEY SIMPLY CANNOT MANAGE BY THEMSELVES... COLLEGE IS HARD ENOUGH!
WHY DO YOU MAKE IT SOUND SO NEGATIVE?

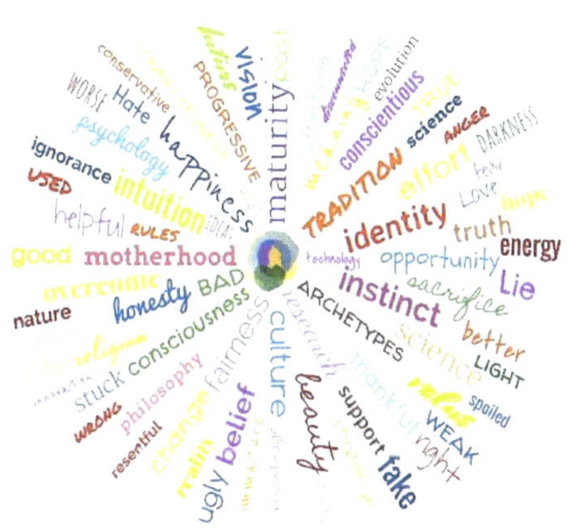
conservative
WORSE
Hate
PROGRESSIVE
VISION
maturity
evolution
conscientious
science
ANGER
DARKNESS
psychology
happiness
ignorance
USED
intuition
TRADITION
effort
Love
helpful
RULES
identity
truth
energy
good
motherhood
technology
opportunity
Lie
instinct
sacrifice
nature
honesty
BAD
ARCHETYPES
better
consciousness
culture
science
LIGHT
stuck
philosophy
fairness
spoiled
WRONG
beauty
support
WEAK
resentful
change
belief
right
ugly
fake

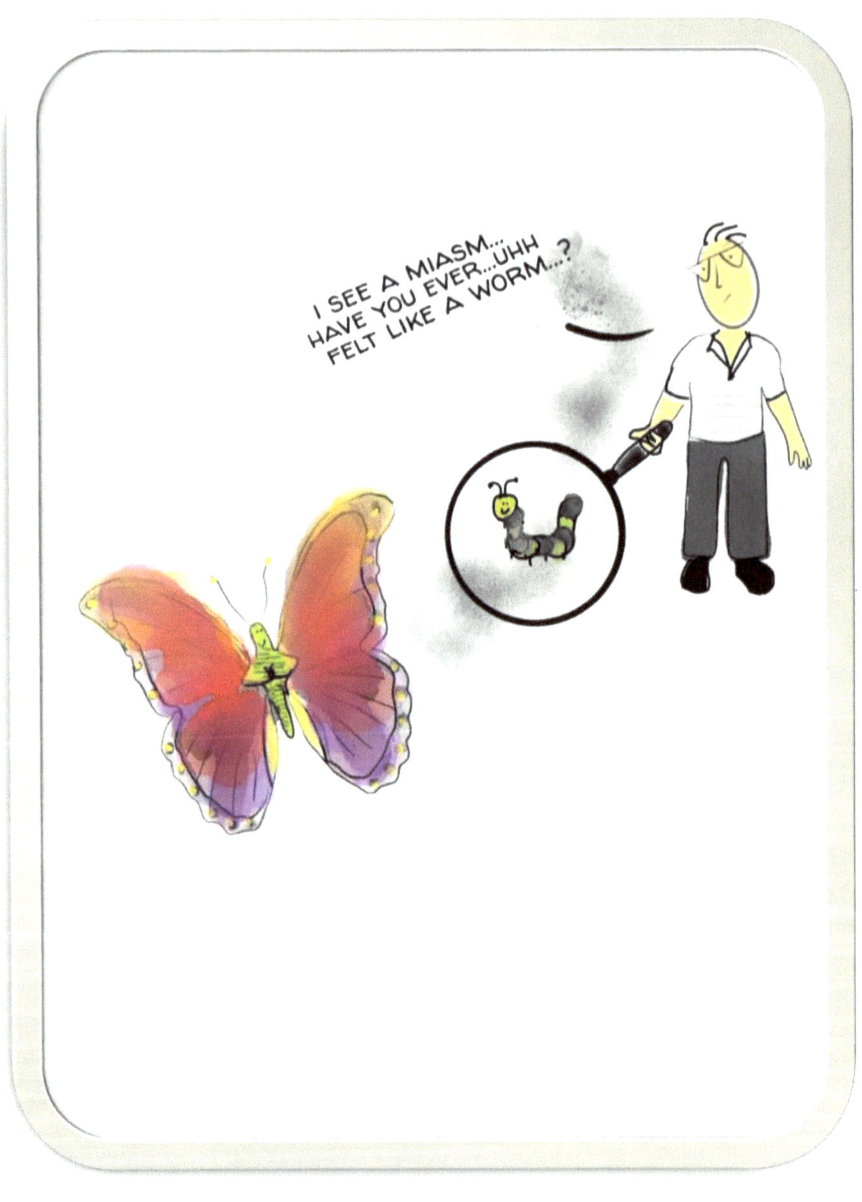
I SEE A MIASM...
HAVE YOU EVER...UHH
FELT LIKE A WORM...?

Suppression and Miasms

By Misna Burelli

But the Devouring Mother syndrome is not just a parental problem. Parents often sense the defenselessness and immaturity of their children, fearing for their survival in a difficult world. It is futile to constantly micromanage our children's every step; nevertheless, the children themselves frequently give us the impression that they are not fully capable of navigating life without our help. They are often immature to the extent of displaying elementary or middle school behaviors when they are in fact almost graduating from high school or even college.[40] What happened?

As mentioned before, the *pulsatilla* archetype presents itself with lots of immaturity. It is a naturally occurring, entirely expected childhood archetype. Almost everyone is likely to own it at some point, as a child. But then the kids get the measles—and with it a good dose of *pulsatilla*—and soon, what has been described above happens: a sense of maturity sets in, preparing children for life, while possibly even preventing future illnesses—or the development of the Devouring Mother expression.

Maybe Mother Nature knows a thing or two about common obstacles on the way to adulthood, trying to provide a mechanism to stimulate appropriate development in children? *Hmmm…*

These are difficult questions. Maybe it follows that we shouldn't suppress measles, but then we also don't like the disease. It's a dilemma. What about just taking the corresponding remedy to avoid it? This is certainly an option and has been explored for about two hundred years in the form of "general prevention of disease".[41] Hahnemann himself was experimenting with the idea of using *belladonna*, another common plant remedy made from deadly nightshade, to prevent scarlet fever, a scary and widespread ailment, at the time. According to his notes, he

---

[40] Neufeld, G. and Mate, G. *Hold On to Your Kids: Why Parents Need to Matter More Than Peers*, Ballantine Books, **2013**

[41] Hahnemann, S. The Cure and Prevention of Scarlett Fever *Lessor Writings* B Jain Publishers, New Dehli

seemed to have had some success with it. Nowadays, some well-known homeopaths call this theory homeoprophylaxis. [42] [43]

By the way, some practitioners have claimed to have seen cases improve after a consultation only—without taking a remedy. Obviously, the necessary energy shift can take place through an adjustment in attitude, just like during psychotherapy. It would be interesting to explore if this shift also happens for physical ailments, thus including all three planes. Maybe, if everyone would work on becoming more mature through therapy sessions or awareness exercises, having the measles would be unnecessary. Could psychotherapy lead to the prevention of measles, or a shift away from the Devouring Mother archetype?

No one would argue that psychotherapy doesn't work, and opening up opportunities for this type of research would clearly be beneficial, but in most cases, it's not enough: remedies work without the psychotherapy part on animals and small children—even many adult cases are just too complex and entrenched in serious physical illness to improve solely by mental energy shift. Besides, people have to be open to the experience, and they need to work on themselves for the shift to occur properly.

But back to suppression: what other common diseases are out there that might have a basis in suppression? How about arthritis? One of the most common remedies to treat influenza is *rhus toxicodendron* (poison ivy), also simply known as *rhus tox*. It treats the kind of flu that comes with body aches, so you can't lay still because everything hurts, but moving your legs just a little bit will make it temporarily better. It helps with this kind of flu and it also treats chronic arthritis.

So, by now the story sounds familiar: are the flu and the remedy the same? Taking the remedy helps with arthritis in many who display a corresponding archetype picture, but would simply "taking the flu" work the same? And what evidence do we have for such a statement?

To make matters more complicated, *rhus tox* is a "universal layer"

---

[42] Birch, K. and Whatcott, C. *The Solution Homeoprophylaxis: The Vaccine Alternative A Parent's Guide to Educating your Child's Immune System* **2012**
[43] Golden, I. *Homeoprophylaxis* Isaac Golden Publications Gisborne Vic. **2004**

remedy,[44] a remedy that is not just a simple archetype picture, but one that is seen universally throughout most human populations. In other words: everyone is susceptible to arthritis and needs some of it. Is that the reason why the flu is constantly circling the globe, always changing shape—so you can pick it up again—but mostly (not always) responding to *rhus tox*?

So just to clarify: what I am saying is that many acute diseases do not produce dangerous miasms—bad imprints with bad outcomes for generations to come—but rather help to clear out those old imprints. And let's not be naïve about this: we all carry them around, those old imprints, some more than others. Clearing them out is protective on a *physical* (for example arthritis), *mental* (for example ADHD) and *emotional* (for example Devouring Mother) level. When we completely refuse to discuss these benefits, ignoring statistics concerning most likely outcomes for the largest part of the population, we might not be doing ourselves a favor. We need to look at what we *miss out* on: some people might statistically be much better off when they *overcome* a little bit of *danger*, especially long-term. Eliminating all adversity from life might have unintended consequences—we humans are known to thrive on challenges.

Is that what Jordan Peterson meant when he said, "you might be winning but you are not growing and growing might be the most important form of winning"? I certainly believe so: optional beneficial challenges should be reintroduced into every person's life.

In times such as ours, with emergency departments everywhere, this could be done in a very controlled environment, where risks can be absolutely minimized. And yes, unfortunately, life does have risks; driving cars is dangerous, and leaving the house exposes us to all kinds of perils, yet we decide to go ahead with it anyway. We do it because we realize that not taking these risks—not driving to a job, and not being a productive member of society—is not a good option. This is so well accepted that no one questions it. So, instead of focusing hysterically on

---

44 Smits, T. *Inspiring Homeopathy: Treatment of Universal Layers,* Emryss Publishers, **2011**

some rare bad outcomes, we just drive to work every day.

The same should be true for medical decisions: we might just as well take some responsibility, have some tests done, and decide if our immune system is ready for a *challenge.* After all, just like going to work, we will get paid for the effort and the risk with the reward of better long-term health.

Math Lesson
Transitive Property of Equality
if measles = pulsatilla
and pulsatilla = Devouring Mom
then Devouring Mom = measles

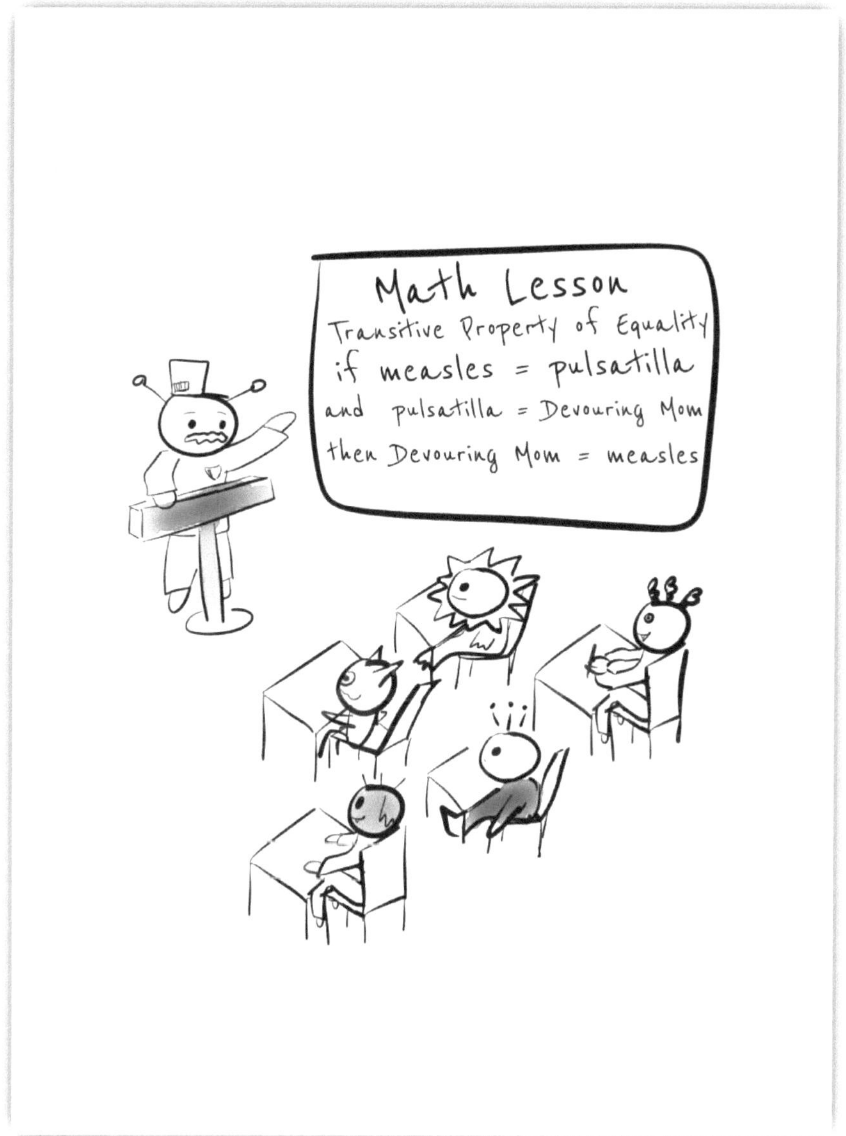

Immune System Lecture Notes

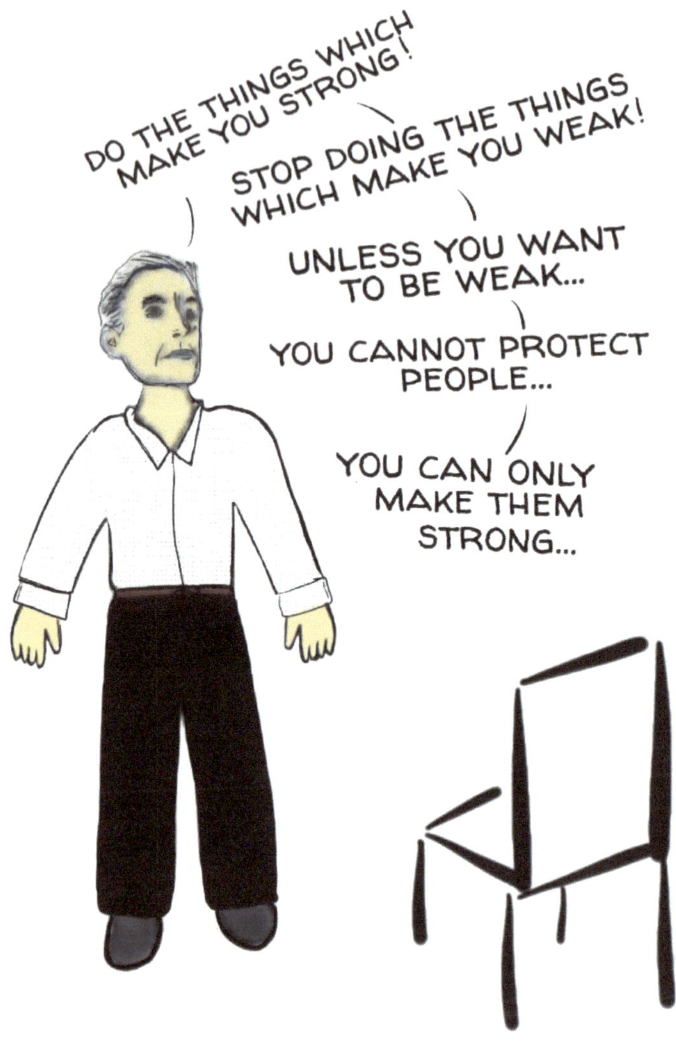
DO THE THINGS WHICH MAKE YOU STRONG!
STOP DOING THE THINGS WHICH MAKE YOU WEAK!
UNLESS YOU WANT TO BE WEAK...
YOU CANNOT PROTECT PEOPLE...
YOU CAN ONLY MAKE THEM STRONG...

Today's lesson: the benefits of battling measles
Jordan Peterson
on difficult learning challenges:
No learning environment is safe, by the way. I don't know about you, but every important thing I have learned in my life was painful.
THESE ARE DIFFICULT CONCEPTS... LET'S HAVE A DISCUSSION!

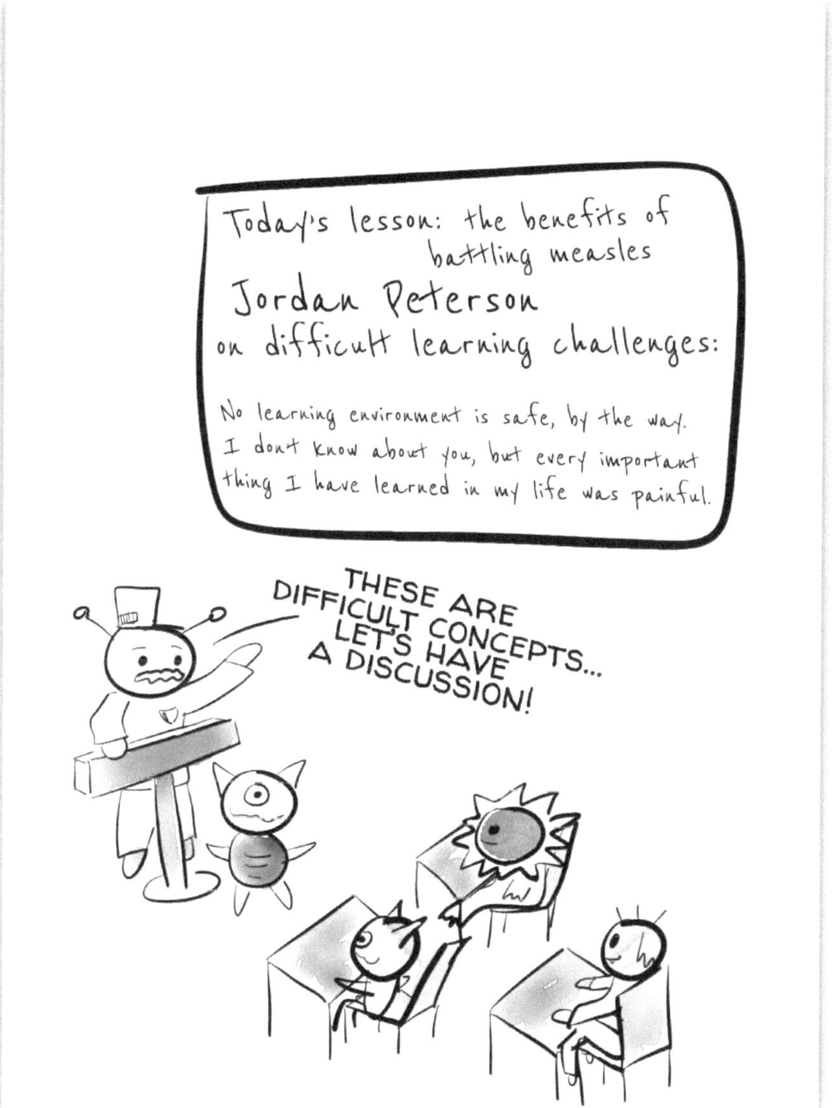

Immune System Lecture Notes

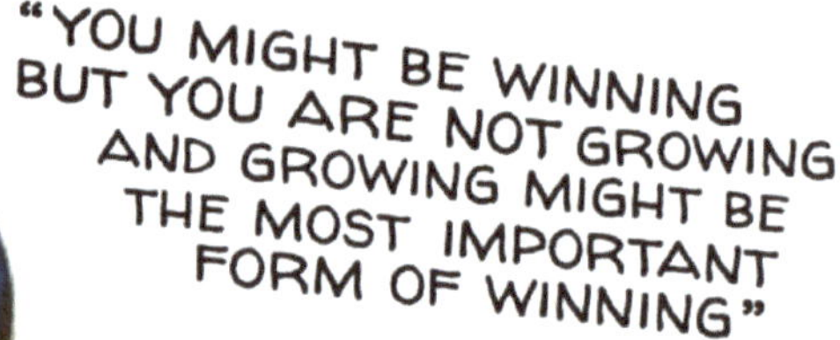
THAT JORDAN PETERSON...
HE'S TAKING WORDS RIGHT
OUT OF MY MOUTH...
LOOK WHAT HE SAID
THE OTHER DAY:
"YOU MIGHT BE WINNING
BUT YOU ARE NOT GROWING
AND GROWING MIGHT BE
THE MOST IMPORTANT
FORM OF WINNING"

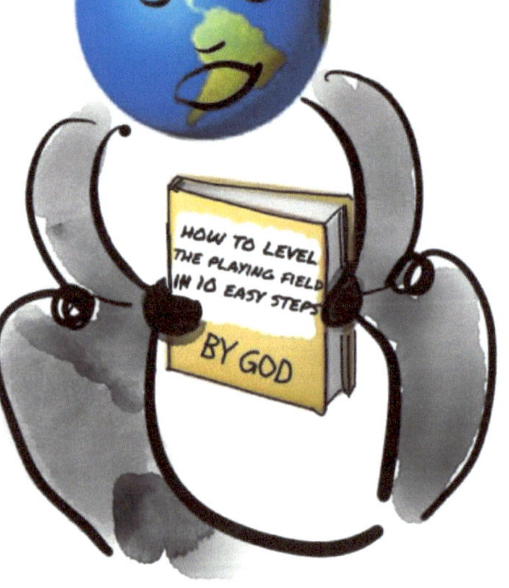
HOW TO LEVEL
THE PLAYING FIELD
IN 10 EASY STEPS
BY GOD

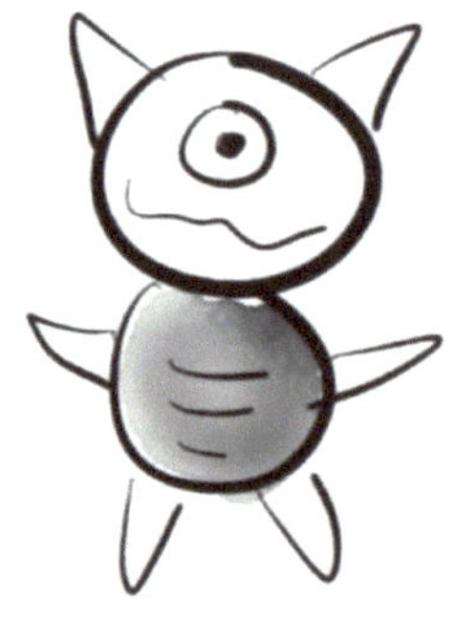

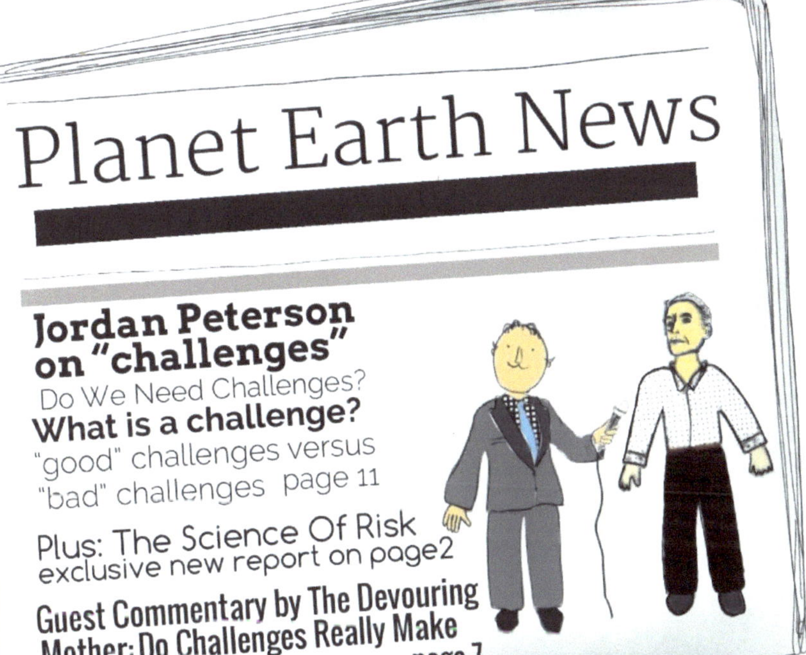
Planet Earth News
Jordan Peterson on "challenges"
Do We Need Challenges?
What is a challenge?
"good" challenges versus "bad" challenges page 11
Plus: The Science Of Risk
exclusive new report on page2
Guest Commentary by The Devouring Mother: Do Challenges Really Make Us Happier?
page 7

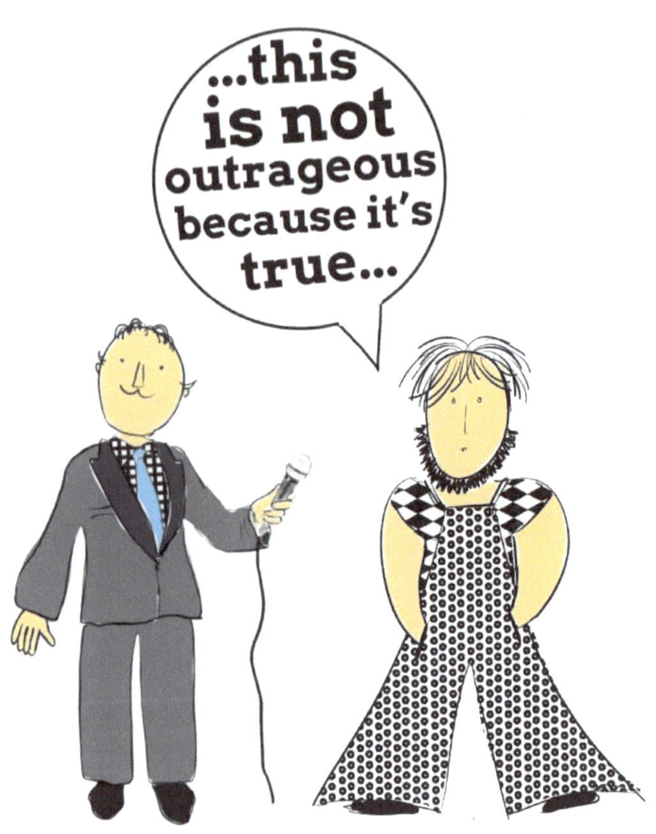
...this
is not
outrageous
because it's
true...

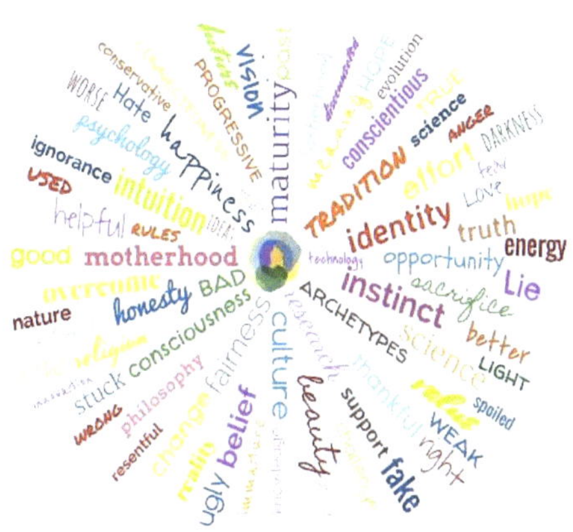
conservative
WORSE
Hate
psychology
happiness
PROGRESSIVE
vision
maturity
evolution
conscientious
science
ANGER
DARKNESS
ignorance
USED
intuition
TRADITION
effort
Love
helpful
RULES
identity
truth
energy
good
motherhood
technology
opportunity
honesty
BAD
instinct
sacrifice
Lie
nature
consciousness
ARCHETYPES
science
better
LIGHT
stuck
philosophy
fairness
culture
beauty
support
spoiled
WEAK
WRONG
resentful
change
belief
ugly
right
fake

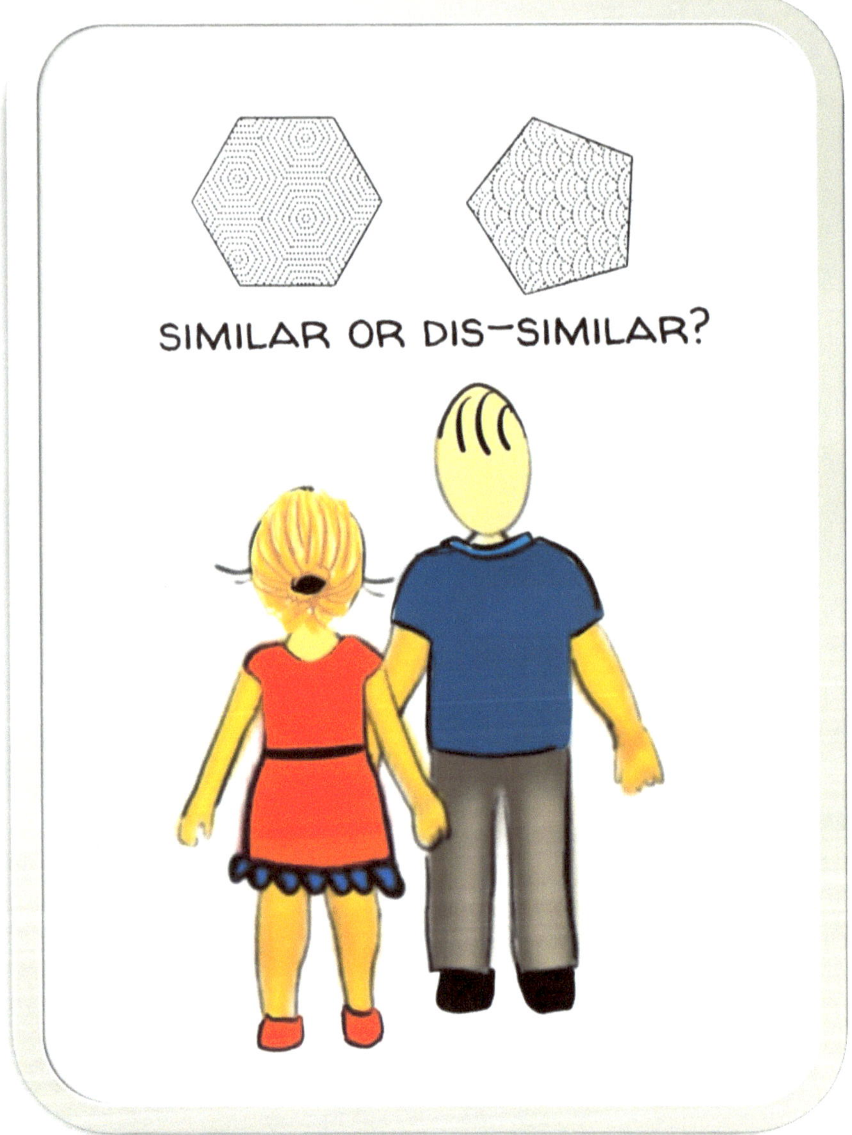
SIMILAR OR DIS-SIMILAR?

Similar and Dissimilar Diseases

By Lena Kratz

I want to emphasize that the statements from the previous section and what follows have not been proven *(yet)* by any scientific method—but have been openly discussed within the homeopathic community. As you can see from previous footnotes, there have been a number of publications—they are not secrets!

The discussion of beneficial "similar diseases" versus detrimental "dis-similar diseases" reaches back to the origins of homeopathy, when, about two hundred years ago, Samuel Hahnemann theorized about it in his book *Organon of Medicine.*[45] He speculated that a disease, which is similar to an ailment, can erase that ailment, thereby improving health, while a dissimilar disease only adds more misery. Even Hippocrates recognized some of these connections by declaring "give me a fever and I can cure any disease". Before the advent of antibiotics, it was common to intentionally infect patients suffering from serious diseases such as syphilis with "lesser" diseases such as malaria to produce a fever—and Hahneman's theory served as the background for this idea.

Getting used to the notion that beneficial diseases indeed exist, the question boils down to this: how do we sort "good" or "bad" diseases into categories, allowing one kind to pass through our bodies, while avoiding the other type at all cost?

There is some literature on this topic, but let's just explore what we already know—it may not be as difficult to answer as it seems: beneficial diseases should mostly be viral in nature. We could go further—some historical chronic disease and cancer treatments have allowed for malaria parasites and strep bacteria as beneficial diseases—but for now, to focus on viruses only leaves us with a much-reduced group of illnesses to work with and less controversy, as we will see in a

---

[45] Hahnemann, S. *Organon of Medicine,* Koethen, Germany, **1810**

minute.[46] [47]

We can distinguish beneficial viral diseases from others by looking at their mortality rate or likelihood of chronic infection. Hepatitis C, B or HIV, for example, are poor candidates—they are dangerous and best avoided. Those diseases also disregard the viral pattern of "you get it once, and it's done"—the self-limiting aspect of acute infections. In addition, they have never been known *traditionally* as "benign childhood diseases", a category made just for viruses such as measles, mumps, rubella and chicken pox. "Benign childhood diseases", used to be a standard component of childhood, alarming no one—did our culture instinctively recognize their importance, and has this knowledge been lost?

Even though they are painted as dangerous and deadly these days, I know *no one* coming to harm through these diseases; none of my older relatives, or even their friends, families and acquaintances—I asked, just to be sure. There are *rare* cases in the population where "benign childhood diseases" left someone disabled or dead. In contrast, I personally know dozens of kids and adults with severe allergies, asthma, autism, learning disabilities, ADHD, depression, burnout, autoimmune diseases and cancer. I also know a number of people dying from car and bicycle accidents! This is just a perspective. How about you? Are you still driving?

The "benign childhood diseases" measles, mumps, rubella and chicken pox fulfill the requirements to be counted among the beneficial diseases—they are short-lived and self- limiting, leading to lifelong immunity. To this list of "benign childhood diseases", I would add the common cold, affectionately called the "drain of the brain" among homeopaths. After all, why do you always get a cold *following* your final exam and why do Alzheimer's patients often *not* suffer from colds anymore? Hopefully this makes you feel better the next time you are "lucky" enough to "catch" a cold, knowing that not everyone is able to

---

[46] Mc Carthy, E.F. The Toxins of William B. Coley and the Treatment of Bone and Soft-Tissue Sarcomas, *Iowa Orthop. J.* **2006**, *26:*154-158

[47] Engelkind, C. Germ of an Idea: William Coley's Cancer-Killing Toxins *Discover Magazine*, **2016**

do so—and that it's just the thing that your immune system ordered. And, of course, let's not forget influenza, although there could be some years where the flu might not be so great. Depending on your immune system, it can be a little bit of a tossup in terms of danger—our damaged immune systems often react poorly these days, allowing secondary *bacterial* infections to occur, leading to the majority of flu deaths.

Generally, in the case of beneficial diseases, we should not be *fighting* Mother Nature; instead we should be working *with* Mother Nature! Rather than being afraid of every fever, sore throat, ear ache or stomach bug—all symptoms the body *created* to get *well*—we should seek out knowledge, in order to give us an understanding of the concept of acute illness. Acute illness is the immune system trying to rid the body of unwanted "stuff"—viruses, leftover metabolic byproducts, toxins and perhaps even "old imprints" aka miasms. All this information is already there for those willing to look!

Finding out how health really works can be scary, especially after coming to the conclusion of being terrified of the wrong thing! There are real threats out there—such as some of the bacterial illnesses we are about to discuss!

If you look at bacterial diseases, they are nothing like "benign childhood diseases", the cold or the flu. Their story is *very* different; there is *no lifelong immunity*. You can come down with strep throat (streptococcus pyogenes) a million times.

This is also why I personally think bacteria-based vaccines such as the DPT have no merit—why vaccinate if you can get it again? The manufacturers of the DPT are fully aware of this shortfall and openly admit that the diphtheria and tetanus vaccines are *not meant* to guard against any microorganisms.[48] They are toxoid vaccines, protecting against the microorganism's toxin. By stimulating a response to the bacterial toxin, our bodies are encouraged to detox faster when we encounter it—it really has *nothing* to do with the invading organism at all.

But to me that is like claiming you can prevent alcohol poisoning

---

[48] https://www.sanofi.us/en/products-and-resources/vaccines

by drinking vodka. Sure, it's totally possible; you can train your liver to detox faster and then down six shots with zero effect. Some college kids are proud of those newly acquired skills, showing them off when coming home for Thanksgiving break. They are really not drunk after those six shots—they got used to the alcohol!

I'm not saying this is a good thing, but it's certainly possible! And it might really have a protective influence against acute alcohol poisoning. But as soon as you stop doing it, the effect will wear off. It's not enough to drink a lot during freshman year and then quit—this is where they tell you to get a "booster" in vaccine language.

Even if valid as a theory—*which it is*—it's a very poor tradeoff destroying your liver in order to be "immune" to alcohol or whatever toxin. If anything, the suspicious "immunity" against toxins is a clear sign that your liver went through a great deal of stress: not exactly a health promoting tactic!

But this is how a toxoid vaccine works, and the diphtheria and tetanus parts of the DPT are toxoid vaccines. They are given to make the body get used to a toxin, a known toxic substance. We should be asking a lot of questions about this practice: what if your liver is unable to deal with this toxin, you suffer from liver disease or you already have a lot of detox problems on your plate?

But even worse, the average person thinks the vaccine protects against the microorganisms, preventing the spread of disease and reducing the danger of outbreaks. Nothing could be further from the truth, because the vaccine is *not meant* to interfere with the microorganism at all. Yet, this supposed protection against spreading is exactly the reason why it has been mandated for school attendance in many places.

So, the diphtheria and tetanus components of the DPT are toxoid vaccines. That leaves the pertussis piece, which is actually made out of disease-causing particles of the Bordetella pertussis bacterium. Although some research shows that previous wild infection with pertussis might produce some natural immunity, there is no guarantee of no other infection occurring down the road. There can't be; this is a *bacterial* disease and, as I explained earlier, you can get those a million times. Even worse, there is indication of colonization of a host with Bordetella pertussis after pertussis vaccination, but the infection is typically asymptomatic. This type of infection *cannot be seen* but it *can be transmitted*, making it impossible to trace the carrier, and health officials know it.[49] Every year many such cases occur with health officials urging more vaccination. Public policy is based on seriously flawed assumptions, and no one is able to correct it.

But back to bacterial infections. They can be nasty every time, with foul smelling mucus and lengthy recoveries. They can be extremely dangerous, and even deadly. Most "flu deaths" occur from secondary bacterial infections. From a homeopathic perspective, bad imprints "miasms" from centuries back generally originated from bacterial diseases and are still causing trouble today. The most prominent ones are syphilis, tuberculosis and gonorrhea. Maybe this century we will add a few more, such as Lyme disease and strep.

Now that we know more about bacterial diseases, it gets easier to understand the difference between similar and dissimilar diseases, and why categorizing measles, mumps, rubella, chicken pox, colds and flus as generally beneficial makes sense. Those viral infections are diseases that we can get only once—colds and flus are new and different every time—and then we possess antibodies.

Is it just a lucky coincidence to develop antibodies after only one exposure, making us immune against further "attacks", or is it because we don't "need" the virus anymore? After all, it did its job, helping us through some transient developmental states, clearing out some toxins and miasms with a temporary rash or a fever—remember Hippocrates: "give me a fever and I can cure any disease".

If you think of these diseases in terms of "needing an illness", your whole attitude about the world shifts, making it clear how Mother Nature has tried hard to develop a *level playing field for everyone*. Maybe your ancestors left you with bad remaining imprints, "miasms", from

---

49 Warfel, J.M. et al. Acellular pertussis vaccines protect against disease but fail to prevent infection and transmission in a nonhuman primate model *Proc. Natl. Acad. Sci. USA* **2014**, *111(2)*: 787-792

previous epidemics? Mother Nature has found a way to reduce the effect: benign childhood illnesses, colds and flus, meant to train the immune system, clearing out some of the bad imprints, and, most remarkably, setting the stage for mental/emotional development, in the form of maturity.

Maybe, if we would allow children to go through beneficial diseases with all the caution and medical support that is appropriate, we could reduce incidents of cancer, strep, heart disease or even AIDS in the future? Wouldn't that be worthwhile exploring?

Two hundred years ago, some researchers thought it was. Using beneficial diseases to treat more serious chronic diseases, or to just give the body a leg up for the future used to be a part of research in medicine.

Some scientists, such as Hahnemann, established this general rule: the *more acute, short-lived* and *self-limiting* a disease, the more likely it is that it is *beneficial.*

But that was a long time ago, and much of that knowledge seems to have been forgotten, except for the fact that measles might protect against cancer. The old research provides a glimpse of where we could be headed if we were willing to look for answers, while accepting the fact that we need an individual risk/benefit analysis for all medical decisions—rather than a one-size-fits-all flowchart mandate.

No wonder healthcare and health insurance costs are through the roof! We are not looking to cure anything, and people are constantly coming back for more. Clearly, *all* medical decisions should be based on *immune system test results*, and beneficial diseases might be allowed to proceed in a controlled environment, among those who are ready for the *challenge,* and with their full consent.

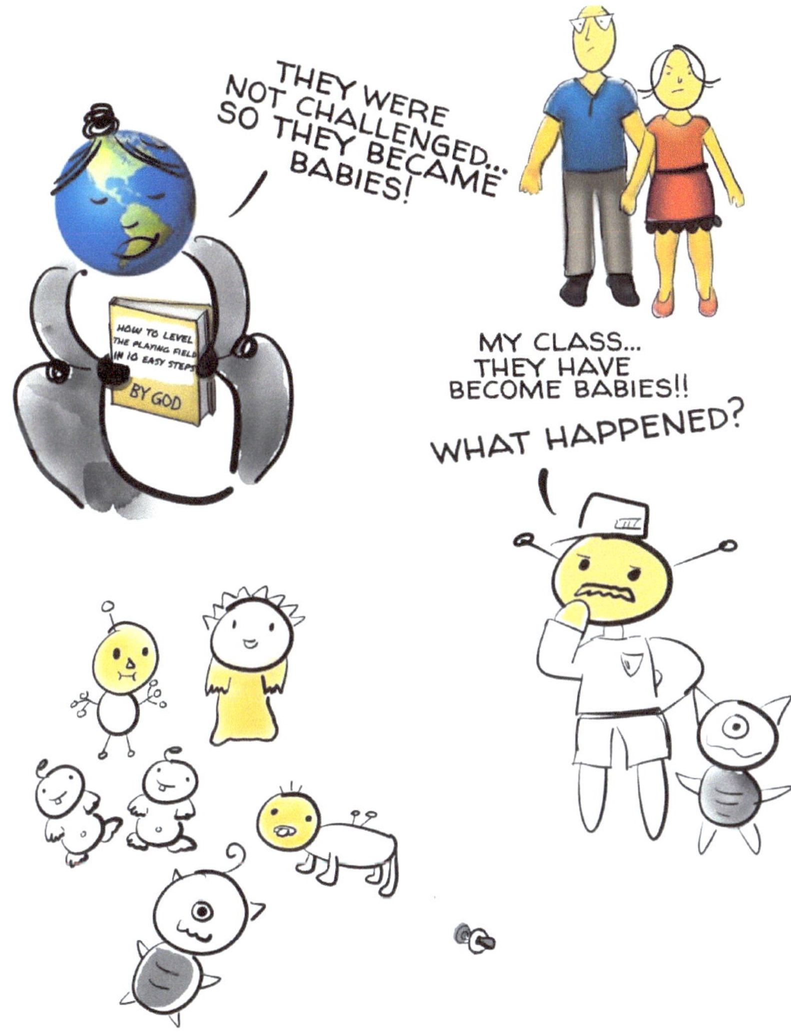
THEY WERE NOT CHALLENGED... SO THEY BECAME BABIES!
HOW TO LEVEL THE PLAYING FIELD IN 10 EASY STEPS
BY GOD
MY CLASS... THEY HAVE BECOME BABIES!!
WHAT HAPPENED?

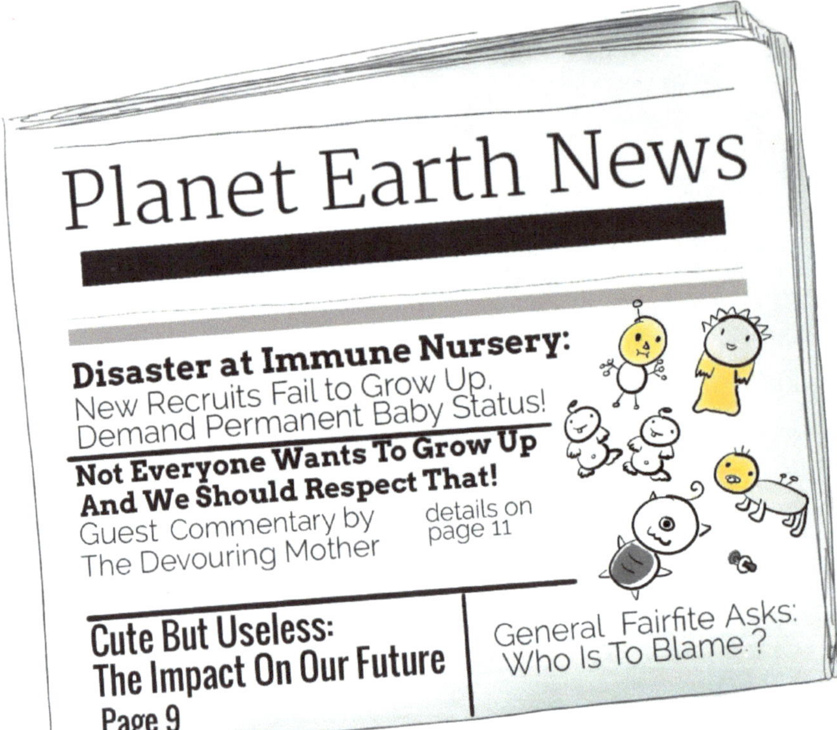
Planet Earth News

Disaster at Immune Nursery:
New Recruits Fail to Grow Up,
Demand Permanent Baby Status!

Not Everyone Wants To Grow Up
And We Should Respect That!
Guest Commentary by
The Devouring Mother
details on page 11

Cute But Useless:
The Impact On Our Future
Page 9

General Fairfite Asks:
Who Is To Blame?

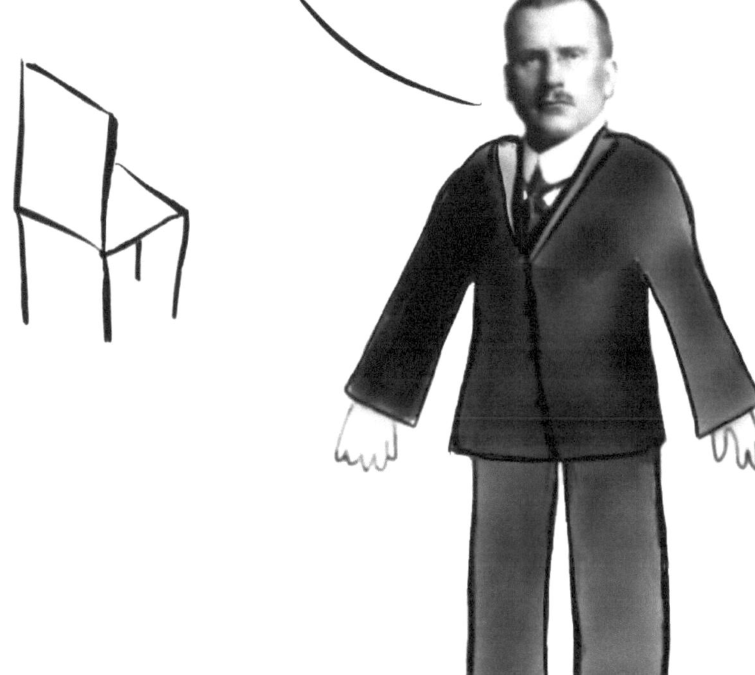
THERE IS NO COMING TO CONSCIOUSNESS WITHOUT PAIN...

BUT HE'S NOT
REALLY DETOXING!!
CONGRATULATIONS...
WHAT NICE DETOXING!!
I'M DETOXING...

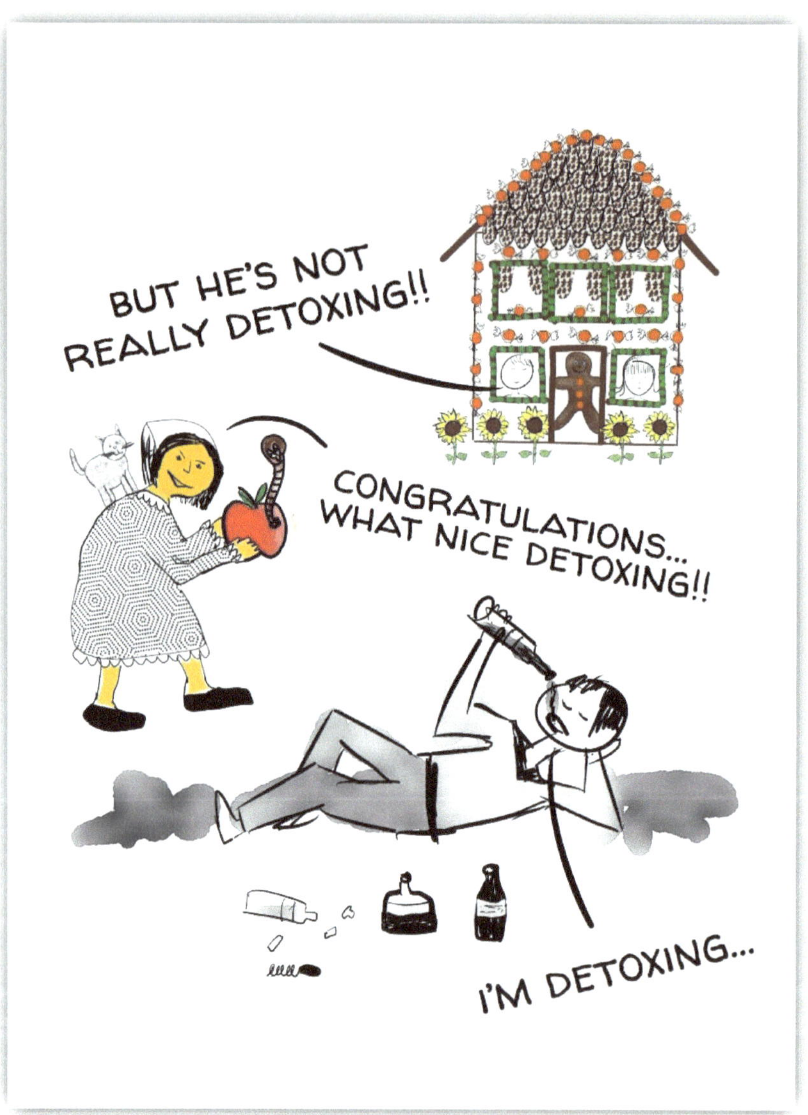

Homeopathic Fairy Tales:
The Emperor's New Clothes

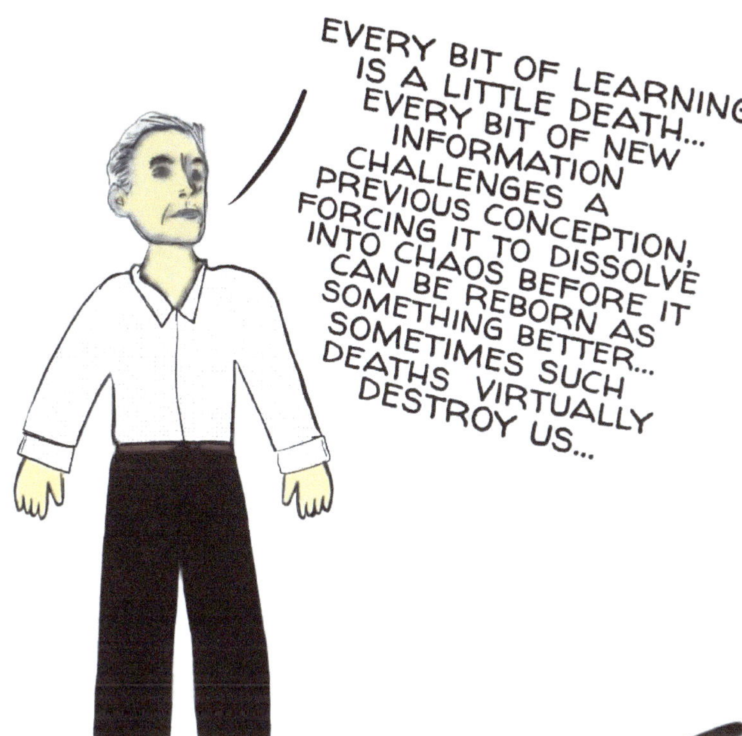
EVERY BIT OF LEARNING
IS A LITTLE DEATH...
EVERY BIT OF NEW
INFORMATION
CHALLENGES A
PREVIOUS CONCEPTION,
FORCING IT TO DISSOLVE
INTO CHAOS BEFORE IT
CAN BE REBORN AS
SOMETHING BETTER...
SOMETIMES SUCH
DEATHS VIRTUALLY
DESTROY US...

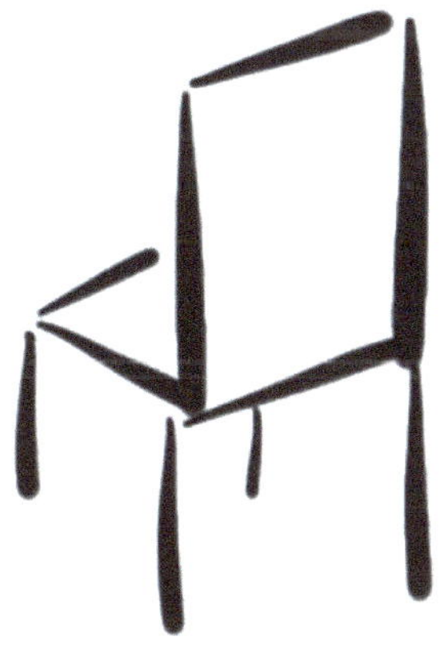

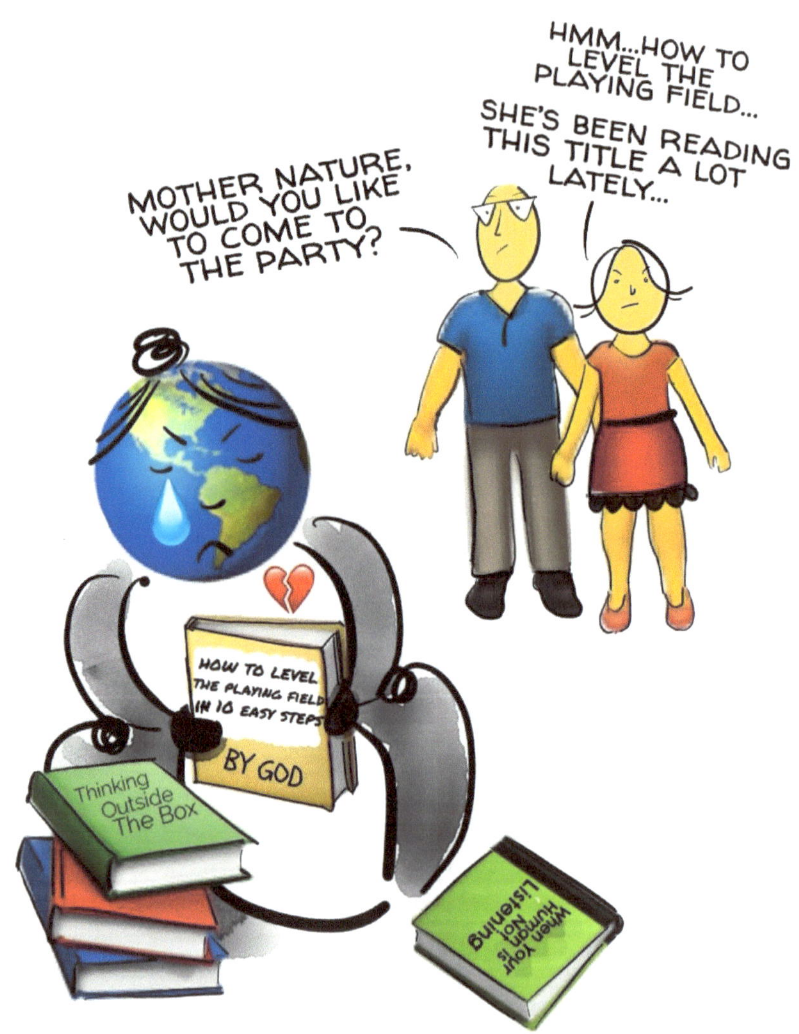
HMM...HOW TO LEVEL THE PLAYING FIELD...
SHE'S BEEN READING THIS TITLE A LOT LATELY...
MOTHER NATURE, WOULD YOU LIKE TO COME TO THE PARTY?
HOW TO LEVEL THE PLAYING FIELD IN 10 EASY STEPS
BY GOD
Thinking Outside The Box
When Your Human is Not Listening

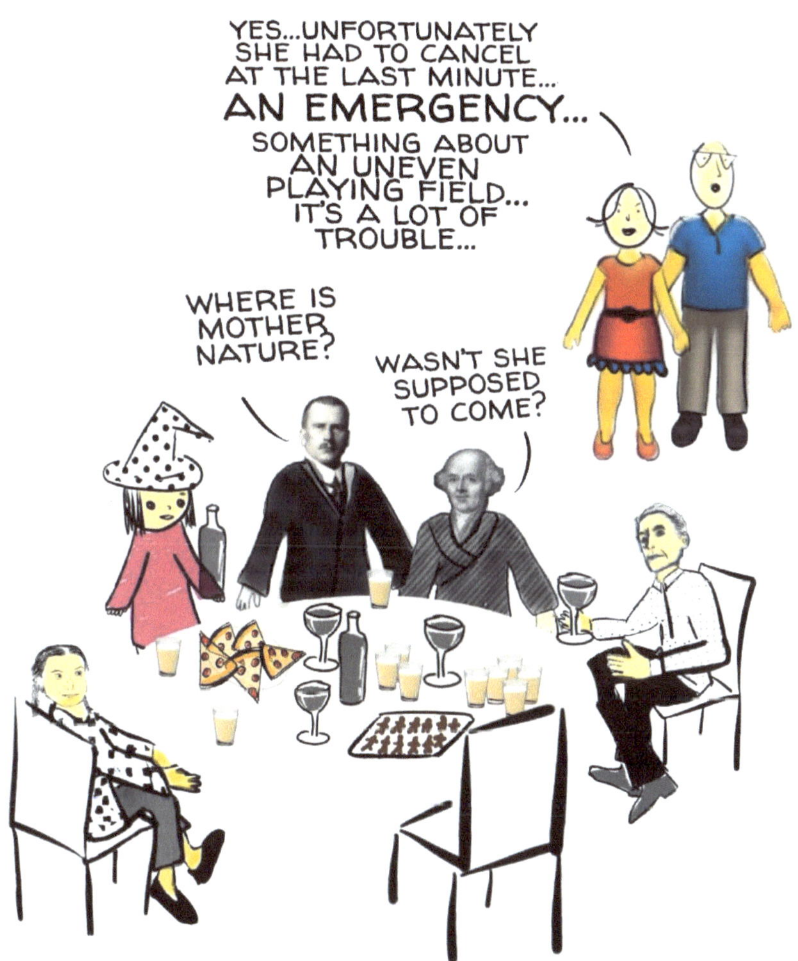
WHERE IS MOTHER NATURE?
WASN'T SHE SUPPOSED TO COME?
YES...UNFORTUNATELY SHE HAD TO CANCEL AT THE LAST MINUTE... AN EMERGENCY... SOMETHING ABOUT AN UNEVEN PLAYING FIELD... IT'S A LOT OF TROUBLE...

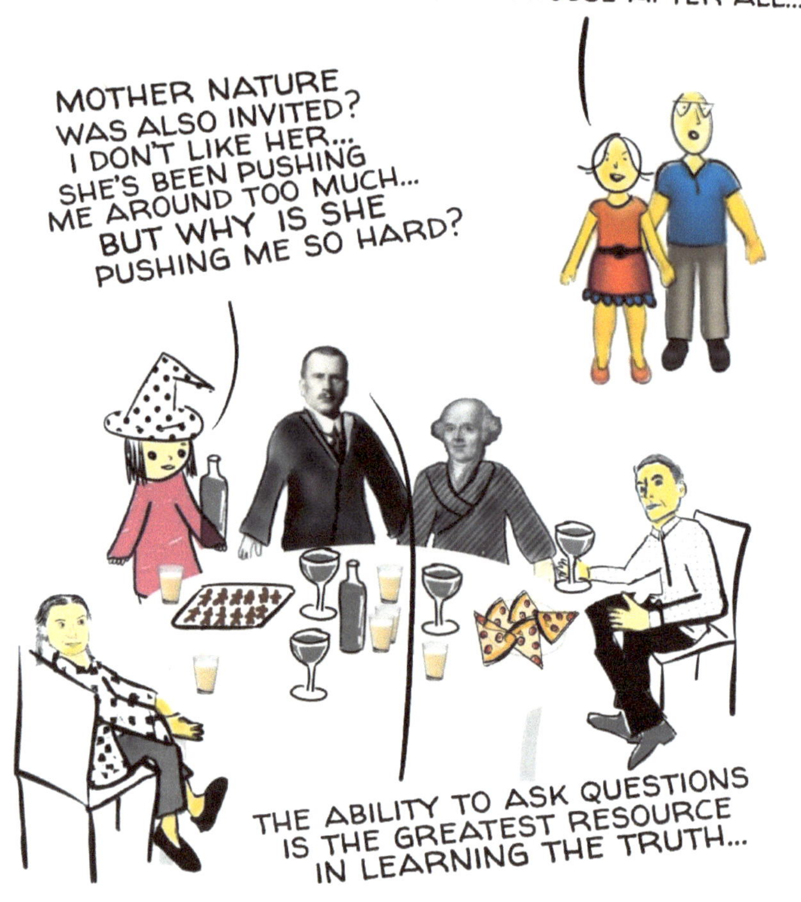
OF COURSE SHE WAS INVITED...
THIS IS HER HOUSE AFTER ALL...
MOTHER NATURE WAS ALSO INVITED? I DON'T LIKE HER... SHE'S BEEN PUSHING ME AROUND TOO MUCH... BUT WHY IS SHE PUSHING ME SO HARD?
THE ABILITY TO ASK QUESTIONS IS THE GREATEST RESOURCE IN LEARNING THE TRUTH...

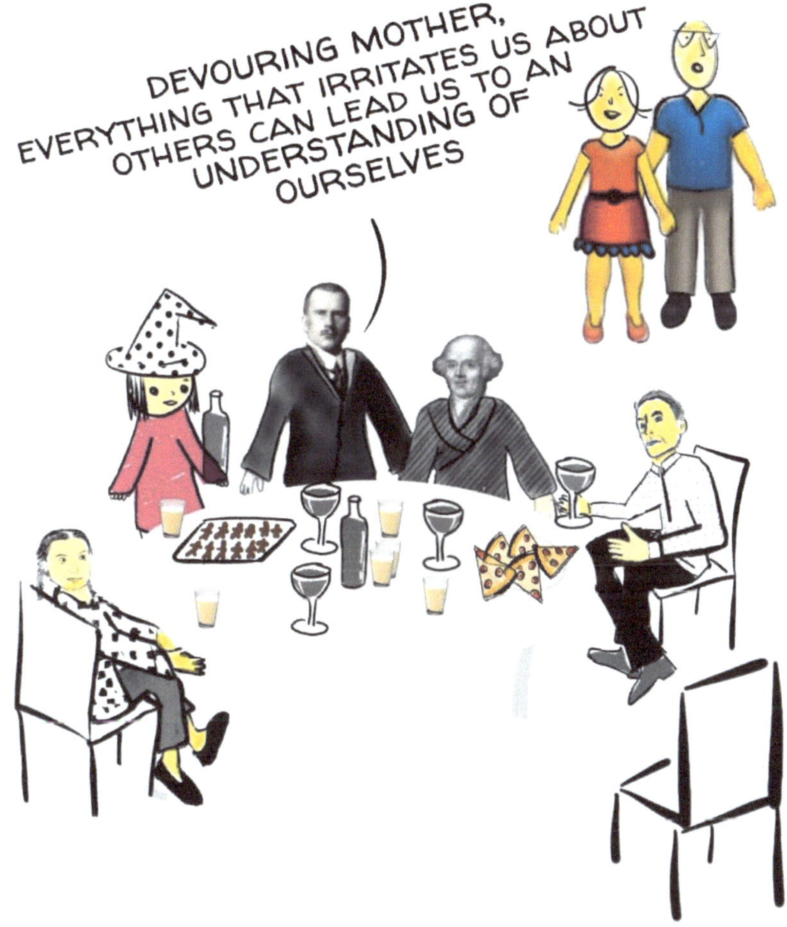
DEVOURING MOTHER,
EVERYTHING THAT IRRITATES US ABOUT
OTHERS CAN LEAD US TO AN
UNDERSTANDING OF
OURSELVES

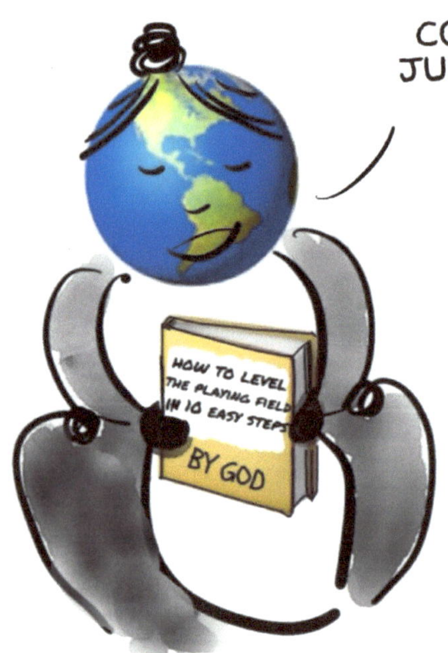
COMMON SENSE IS
JUST AN EXPRESSION
OF BALANCE
HOW TO LEVEL
THE PLAYING FIELD
IN 10 EASY STEPS
BY GOD

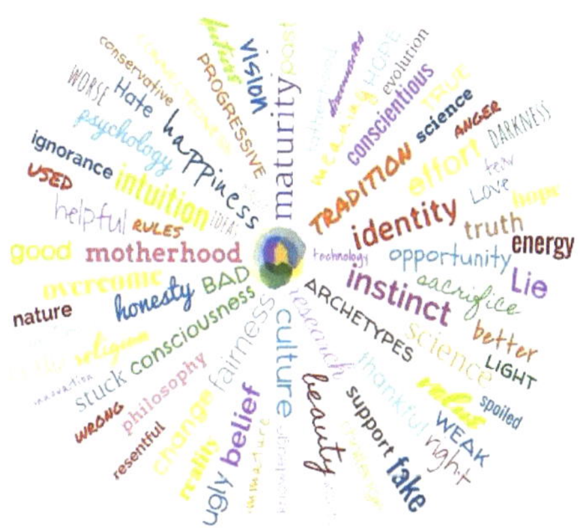
conservative
WORSE
Hate
psychology
happiness
PROGRESSIVE
VISION
maturity
evolution
conscientious
science
ANGER
DARKNESS
ignorance
USED
intuition
TRADITION
effort
Love
helpful
RULES
identity
truth
energy
good
motherhood
technology
opportunity
Lie
BAD
instinct
sacrifice
honesty
nature
consciousness
ARCHETYPES
science
better
LIGHT
culture
religion
stuck
fairness
research
philosophy
beauty
thankful
values
spoiled
WRONG
support
WEAK
change
belief
right
resentful
reality
fake
ugly

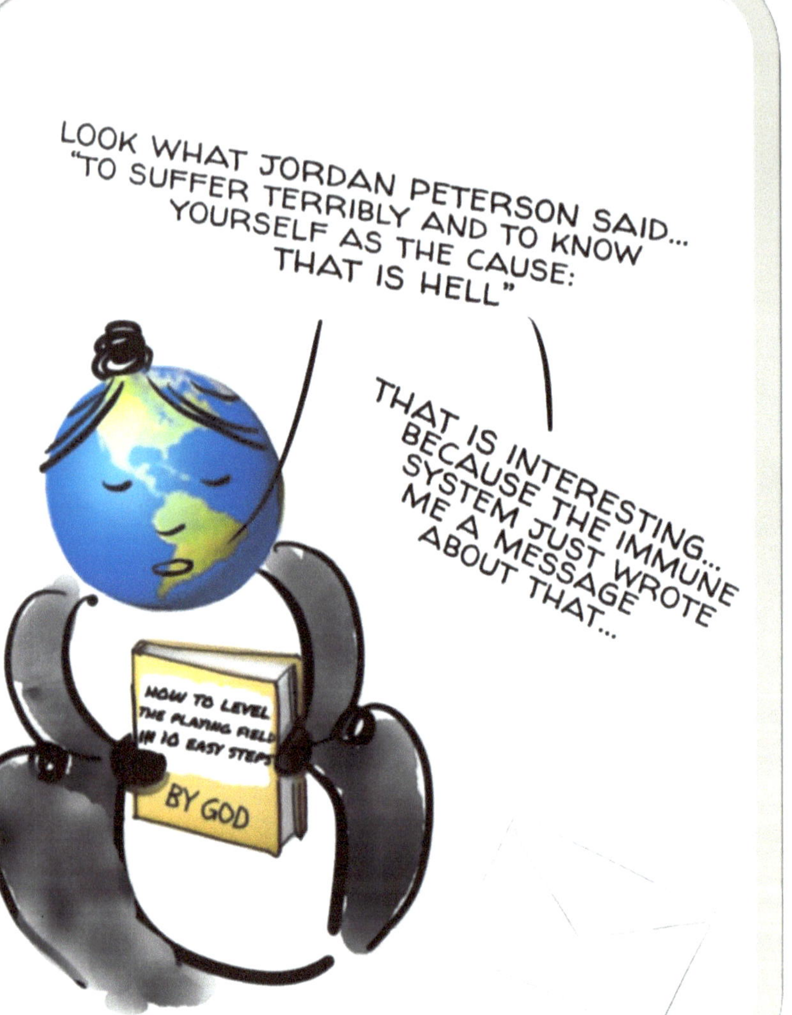
LOOK WHAT JORDAN PETERSON SAID...
"TO SUFFER TERRIBLY AND TO KNOW YOURSELF AS THE CAUSE: THAT IS HELL"
THAT IS INTERESTING... BECAUSE THE IMMUNE SYSTEM JUST WROTE ME A MESSAGE ABOUT THAT...
HOW TO LEVEL THE PLAYING FIELD IN 10 EASY STEPS
BY GOD

A Message from the Immune System
By Misna Burelli

When we are sick, we start worrying about our immune system. Is it too weak? Should we try boosting it with vitamins, herbal supplements or cold showers? Or is it working too hard, giving rise to allergies? Or both? Would that even be possible, and what's the difference? How *does* the immune system work?

I learned some of the most interesting details about the immune system from a biology class. It was easily one of the best classes I have ever taken. Who could have predicted the joy that comes with watching such a beautiful system in action, observing the million little things that make it work—*simply fascinating!*

The lecture went a little bit like this: ...so here are some of the components of your immune-system-army detecting some invaders and calling on the whole body to declare an emergency. The defense is blasting the intruders—just to be on the safe side—carefully digesting them into small pieces and then mounting them onto transport modules. This way they can send messages to even the last corners of the system to be on the lookout for this type of trespasser. Upon contact, immune system personnel has been instructed to immediately neutralize any such invaders, while reporting the incident to the nearest defense checkpoint—preparing for serious battle! The defense department implements all these plans with exact precision, leaving no doubt that all commands are followed in record time, while also making sure to absolutely avoid any incidents of friendly fire. Yes, the immune system works like an army—an army that is at the center of every human, giving its all to protect us!

The two main complimentary branches of the immune system are the humoral and the cell-mediated immunity, each working to fulfill their individual tasks in ways that support the body as a whole. Considering its unbelievable complexity and flawless design, I won't get into any more details here, except to say that, when I started thinking about my hay fever symptoms, I suddenly realized that they were *impossible*. There was absolutely *no way* for hay fever to just casually develop out of nowhere, or perhaps because my environment was "too clean" or "too dirty". It was way too unlikely, due to the extreme precision and reliability that was built into the immune system—it wouldn't be knocked over by something as simple as a clean house. Yet, it was obvious that I did, in fact, have hay fever—what had happened?

As outlandish as it sounds, it seems likely that my immune system actions were based on false information, violating standard immune system protocol. It became clear that something, or someone, must have taught my immune system the specifics of attacking pollen, intentionally trying to confuse it and preventing it from working right. It must have been a trick of some sort, as human immune systems employ a million feedback loops, authentication codes, and confirmation processes—every student's head was spinning while learning about it!

It is very obvious that allergies should never happen, and the same is true for the other version of immune system "mistake", the autoimmune response. The amount of careful planning that prevents this type of thing from happening, to a healthy body, is mind boggling. It simply would not happen for no reason.

And yet, both of these scenarios occur *frequently* these days! I almost don't know anyone anymore without either an allergy or an autoimmune condition. So, if it is that difficult to mess with the immune system, then why does it happen?

To make matters worse, another dangerous condition is on the rise as well. In this case, the body allows foreign-looking cells to proliferate uncontrollably. If you study the literature explaining the growth of the placenta during pregnancy, and the whole idea that a new life—a foreign organism—is allowed to survive in the womb, it becomes clear that it must be deliberate. The immune system is deliberately accommodating the baby and the invading placenta, switching off probably more than a million buttons to make it possible.[50] And it

---

[50] Gonzalez, N.J. and Isaacs, L.L. *The Trophoblast and the Origins of Cancer*, New Spring Press, New York, **2009**

should! Obviously, it is worth it to have an altered immune response during pregnancy—otherwise human life would be impossible! But what would make an immune system switch off these one million buttons in order to accommodate a tumor? We expect it to know better! It seems like someone messed with the chain of command, giving a totally irrational order, originating from high up in the immune system control tower, overriding all common sense!

Just like in the case of allergies and autoimmune diseases—attacking pollen or body tissues—the immune system is totally confused. In fact, it is even worse than simple confusion, it looks more like *polarization*: either it attacks everything, or it doesn't attack at all.

So how is all this possible?[51] Before we try to answer this question—and yes, *suppression* of all kinds is certainly one of the culprits—let's briefly go back to our archetypal pictures and their connections to epidemic diseases. During outbreaks, we often see the related pictures emerge as a cultural quirk or Zeitgeist. Some well-known examples include the tuberculosis (*tuberculinum*) stereotype who is creative, productive, restless, easily bored, aggressive, angry, even violent, "burns the candle on both ends", slightly OCD, likes to travel, is eternally unsatisfied, and so on. Or the gonorrhea (*medorrhinum*) one who is a night owl, is always in a hurry, frequently loves the ocean and tends to be, "a little on the wild side", having too much fun.

These are symptoms from the emotional planes of the disease outbreaks, and they can affect an entire society, if enough people come down with a specific illness.

We, as a society, have definitely recently been sick enough to earn a few new badges in our game of creating brand-new archetype images—21st century archetype images! But how do they look like, and how do they fit in with our other "basic" archetypes? Would the Devouring Mother still be recognizable, under these new badges? Because that is what happens frequently—archetypes overlap, confusing the picture. Tuberculosis, for example, could overlie a personal

[51] Fraser, H. *The Peanut Allergy Epidemic: What's Causing It And How To Stop It* Skyhorse, Third edition, **2017**

constitutional archetype, making it harder to recognize both pictures. A good homeopath knows this, and will attempt to either give two remedies, or find something that addresses both personalities.

However, recently, some homeopaths from around the world, especially from India, where homeopathy plays a large role in public healthcare, have expressed concerns that there are too many interferences in everyday archetype pictures! An atmosphere of disbelief permeates some of these conversations, such as, "I have no idea what happened to you Americans. In my country, most of the archetypes I see in my clients are so clear. I use predominantly polychrests—the most common, most well-known remedies—with great results. But here, all I see is confusion".

That's exactly where the problem is: here in the US, it used to be just as easy, but these days, many homeopaths can't find clear pictures any more. There are very few textbook examples for archetype selection, often making the art of homeopathy into a frustrating endeavor. Disease states have become so deep and entrenched, leading to one disorder placed on top of another, that many practitioners now start their clients on general detox remedies first. And if they are lucky, after seeing some improvements in their clients, a clearer picture will eventually emerge.

As mentioned in the beginning, good results from homeopathy depend on getting the archetype right—otherwise there will be *no* results. But if there is too much overlap between pictures, the archetype is too difficult to find, resulting in limited success.

Is that what happens to many people when they first try homeopathy—their cases are too difficult for real progress to occur? *Probably!*

But what is this new archetype which is overlapping everything and making the process of remedy selection so challenging? That's the all-important question we will try to tackle in the next chapter. Just be prepared: it's a message from the immune system!

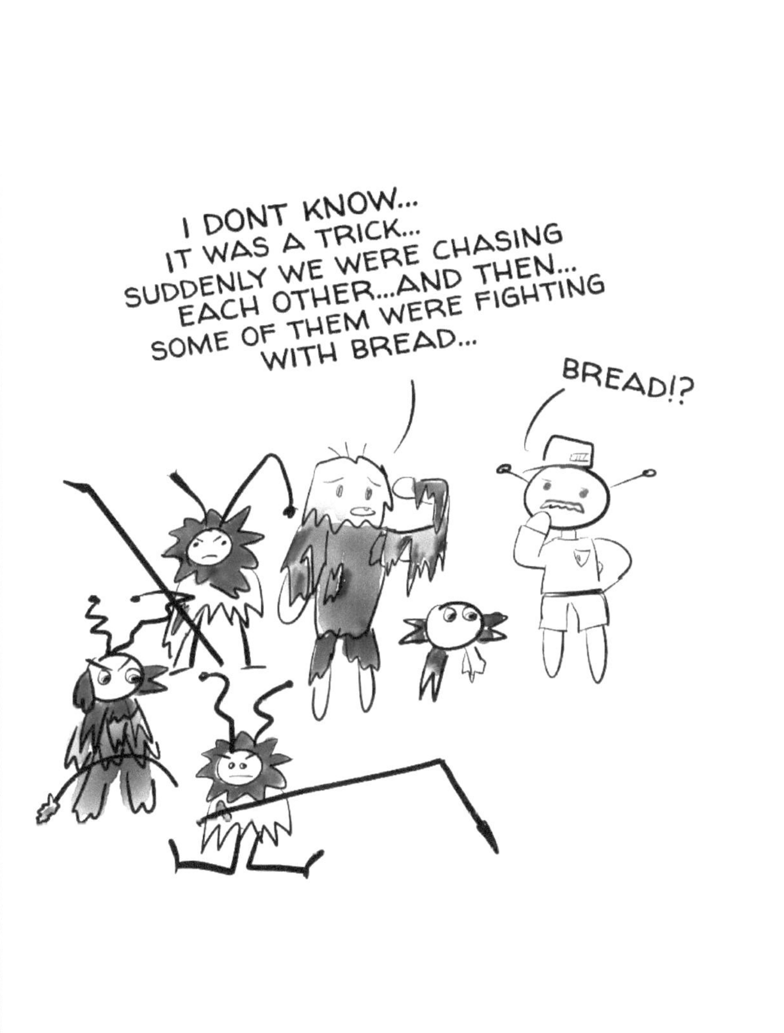
I DONT KNOW...
IT WAS A TRICK...
SUDDENLY WE WERE CHASING
EACH OTHER...AND THEN...
SOME OF THEM WERE FIGHTING
WITH BREAD...
BREAD!?

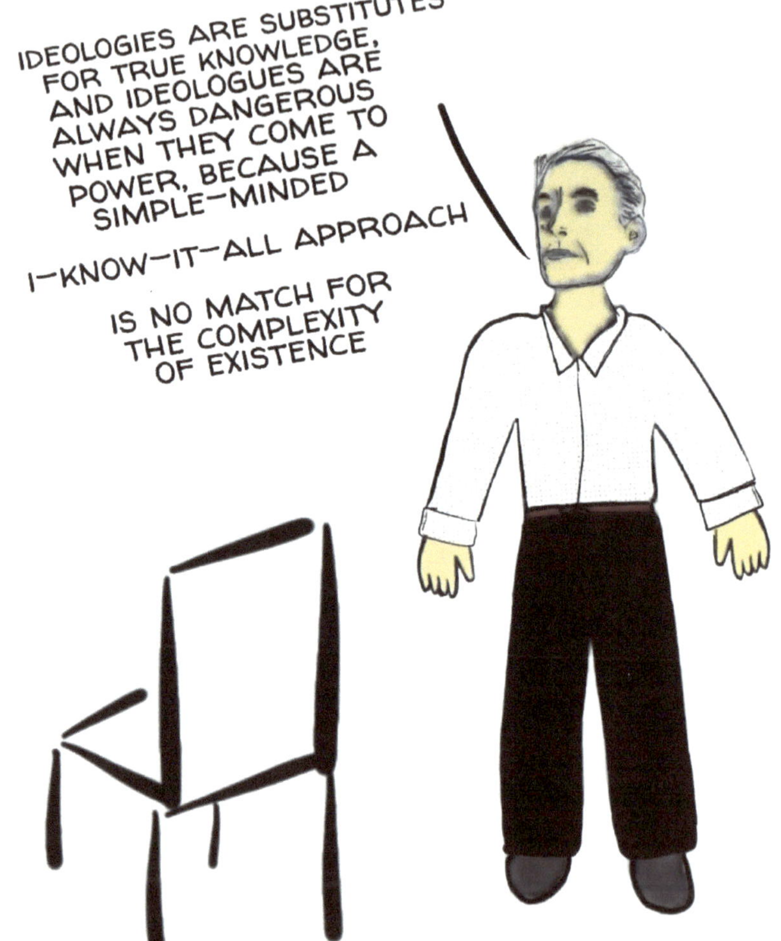
IDEOLOGIES ARE SUBSTITUTES FOR TRUE KNOWLEDGE, AND IDEOLOGUES ARE ALWAYS DANGEROUS WHEN THEY COME TO POWER, BECAUSE A SIMPLE-MINDED
I-KNOW-IT-ALL APPROACH
IS NO MATCH FOR THE COMPLEXITY OF EXISTENCE

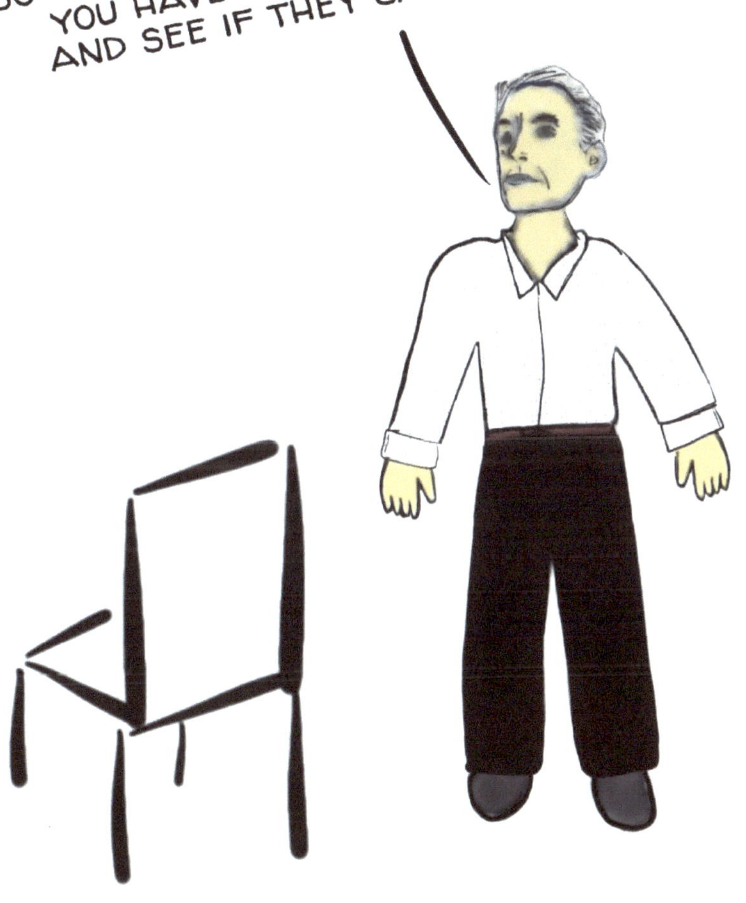
ALMOST ALL IDEAS ARE WRONG...
SO TACKLE THEM WITH EVERYTHING
YOU HAVE IN YOUR ARSENAL
AND SEE IF THEY CAN SURVIVE

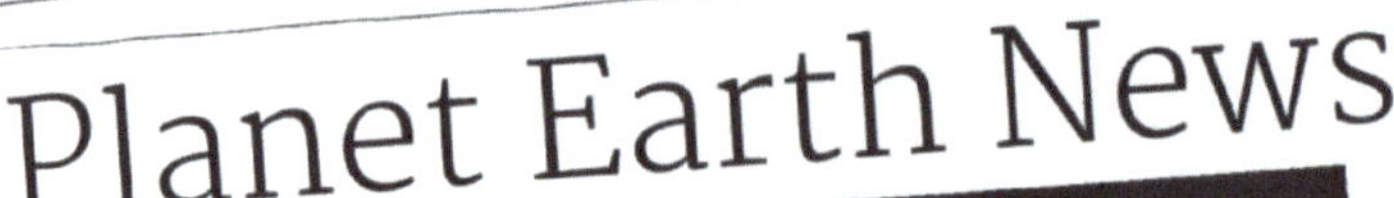

Planet Earth News

General Fairfite not happy: claims immune system has been tricked! page 3

Big Questions: How Can You Trick The Immune System? page 5 Our Experts Discuss

"Fake Enemies"...Do They Exist? A Conversation With Al Ehrgy
Go To Page 7 For Details

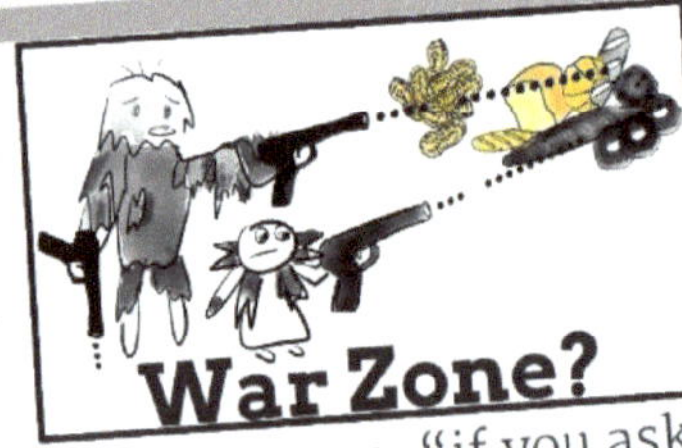

Veteran: "if you asked me 10 years ago to fight peanuts I would have called you crazy..."

"Now they do it all the time!"

War Inside The Body! page 10

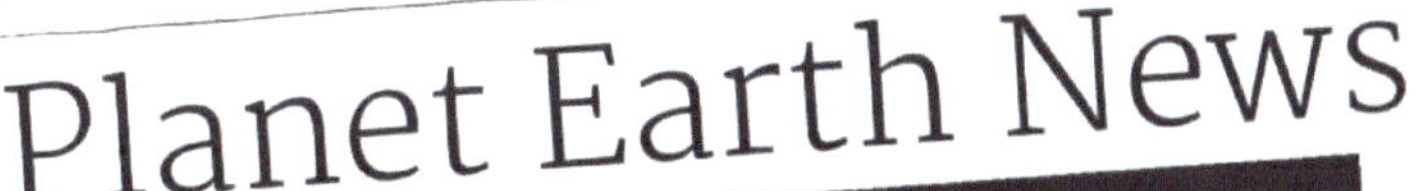

Planet Earth News

Are Humans Unappreciative?

Interview With Mother Nature: Humans Don't Care About Missing Out, Obsessed With Risk

Full Discussion On Page 3

Fact Check: Is It True?

Things You Cannot See: Mother Nature's Attempt at Equal Opportunity page 5

How Large Are Modern Playing Fields? We asked football players- here is their answer! page 10

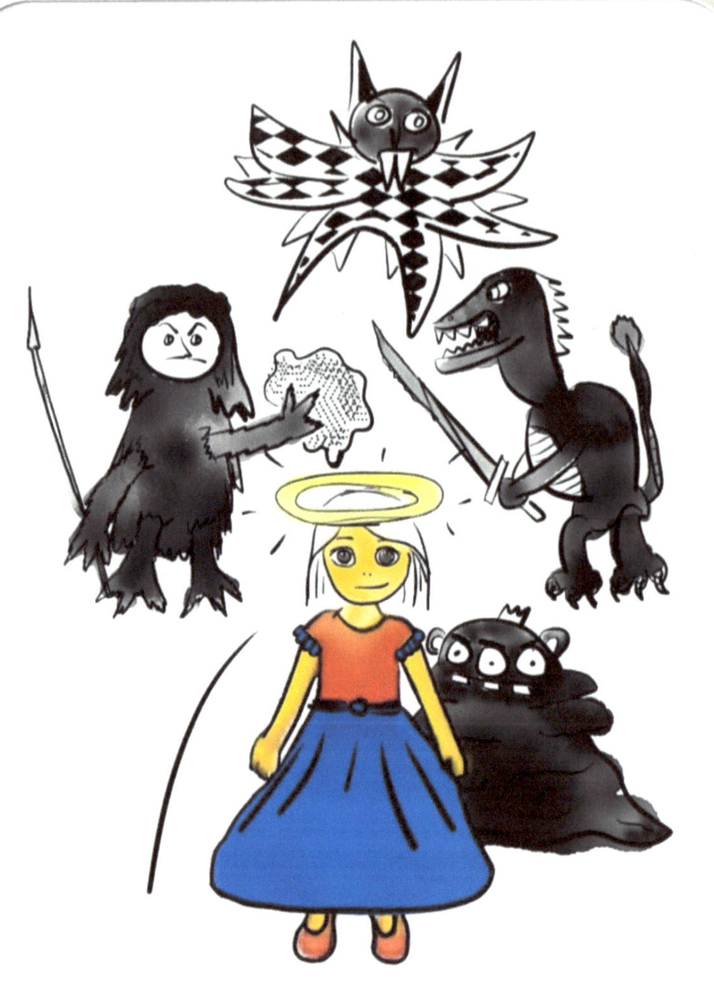
I DO BELIEVE THAT EVERYONE IS GOOD...
SO GLAD THERE IS ONLY GOODNESS OUT THERE!

Our Polarized Immune Systems as Archetypes

By Lena Kratz

So, let's play a little quiz game: imagine a disease that is called *Immune-confusion*. Based on its physical symptom presentation, you are supposed to predict its mental/emotional archetype picture or, in other words, how the disease looks like on the second and third planes. Remember: mental/emotional symptoms mirror physical symptoms in their expression of the underlying pathology. Let's get started.

…………….

Immune-confusion 001: most of the victims of this disease suffer from an ailment called an allergy, which is a physical presentation of an unwarranted immune system attack against harmless entities in the environment. The illness is common.

Predicted Emotional Archetype: it is not too far-fetched to conclude that the emotional archetypal picture of this disease could consist of the following: severe aggressive behavior, aggression toward innocent bystanders and even friends, aggression that is unexplained and has no reason. Being triggered by things that should not upset anyone and being in constant combat mode, while having no one to fight with. Is this the basis for "snowflake syndrome"?

…………….

The next disease is called *Immune-confusion 002*: most of the victims of this disease suffer from an ailment called autoimmunity, which is a physical presentation of an unwarranted immune system attack against the self.

Predicted Emotional Archetype: in this case, the emotional archetypal picture of the disease could include self-destruction: self-harm, depression, self-hate and suicidal thoughts.

....

And then there is *Immune-confusion 003*: this one is tricky. Most of the victims of this disease have their body growing an almost identical part of itself, but with dysfunctional mitochondria, the energy producing parts of the cell. Doctors have been unable to find a reason for this to happen. Yes, the growth is a tumor, and the disease is called cancer. Depending on how the disease progresses, the tumor might take over the whole body and kill its host, all while the immune system is sitting there watching idly. An immune system problem is again at the root of the disease: the immune system is unresponsive.

Predicted Emotional Archetype: in this case the emotional archetypal picture includes an unreasonable desire to help and please everyone, no matter how undeserving they might be, or what the resources are. Ruthless and cruel people might take over, but no one in charge realizes that. No alarms go off. Actually, the alarms and defenses have all been disabled and walls have been ripped apart. Confusion of identity linked with a weak ego and low self-confidence are primary emotional indicators. This case is not like the first two cases, having the immune system attack the wrong thing. In this case the immune system gave up. It quit. It was looking—but it couldn't see anything wrong. This is the state you get when people claim they don't know what evil is. They really mean it. They are not pretending. They just can't see anything bad in the world. Not in themselves and not in others. They are simply too nice for their own good. Often, kids like this with "unsecure emotional borders" are mercilessly teased and bullied in school because everyone else can sense their defenselessness and their naïve nature. The extreme polarity is noticeable in this archetype—there is no negative pole. The balance is off.

This is the emotional state of cancer, a well-known archetypal picture, which has a lot of application in today's world. Just to be clear here: real physical cancer is the end stage of a journey that often starts with these archetypal emotional pictures, which begin years, if not decades, ahead of what we call the disease of cancer. Sadly, these days, the archetype with its weak defenses on the physical, emotional and mental plane is often obvious in children even.[52] Just to clarify—not all cancer automatically fits this archetype picture, there are some cancers that develop differently and have other emotional pictures.

....

How about one more? *Immune-confusion 004*: most of the victims of this disease suffer from a range of physical ailments, including stomach pains, diarrhea, constipation, infections of all kinds, allergies and general metabolic problems. The physical symptoms are unclear and all over the place. Patients experience sleeping problems. The disease expresses itself mostly on the mental/emotional level, making the picture we are looking for identical to the disease—it *is* the mental/emotional archetype, needing no prediction. The disorder occurs on a spectrum, with some people being really smart and even extremely talented, while others are cognitively disabled and unable to achieve academically. Some of the more severe cases include children who have trouble with toilet training and language development. They often cannot speak in sentences, even as teenagers. Frequently they avoid eye contact, looking inward onto themselves, without interacting with the greater world out there—as if they couldn't see over the border. They are socially awkward; they avoid social interactions and have no friends. They often don't know what a "friend" is, or an "enemy", "themselves" or "others". They don't know danger. They often come up closely to other people's faces, violating their personal spaces without noticing. They seem not to know where they end in space—where their proper borders are. The official name of the disease is autism.

....

---

[52] Mueller, M. The Cancer Diathesis *The American Homeopath, Vol 16*, **2010**

How do I know that autism is an immune system disease and not just a freak DNA mutation or inherited disability as is often claimed? Well, how about this: after spending about 200-280 million dollars yearly on autism research,[53] focusing mostly on behavioral approaches and genetics, there have been absolutely *no* results in terms of a prevention or a cure![54] At the same time, many personal autism cure accounts have been published, showing that autistic children *can* and *do* benefit from immune supporting interventions.[55] I'm not saying that genetic variations could never play any role in the onset of autistic behavior, but let's just be honest about two things: First, there are no genetic epidemics—and autism is becoming a major health emergency of epidemic proportions—and second, immune system interventions, including a switch to a strict diet, work wonders for many autistic children.[56]

And the same is true for the other three immune-confusion illnesses above.[57] The main cause, the underlying pathology, for these diseases is found in *immune system damage*.[58]

Which brings us back to our original questions: Are these disease states responsible for the unexpected archetype overlaps? Is the culprit simply general immune system damage? How could this be so prevalent in our society right now—shouldn't our very expensive healthcare system prevent such outcomes?

The trouble with healthcare is that we don't recognize the *general process*, the *principle* behind disease as a whole. All illnesses have more in common with each other—are more related to each other than our

---

53 https://report.nih.gov

54 https://www.washingtonpost.com/education/2018/12/13/huge-issue-that-most-funding-autism-research-ignores

55 Conroy, H. et al. *The Thinking Moms' Revolution: Autism beyond the Spectrum: Inspiring True Stories from Parents Fighting to Rescue Their Children*, Skyhorse Publishing, **2013**

56 Lyons-Weiler, J. *The Environmental and Genetic Causes of Autism*, Skyhorse Publishing, **2016**

57 Joyner, M.J. What Happens When Underperforming Big Ideas In Research Become Entrenched? *JAMA* **2016** *316(13):* 1355-1356

58 Keogh, L. Why it may be time to reconsider the money spent on genetics research *The Conversation* March 1, **2017**

current medical model allows. We can't find a cure by handing out a pill for every disease on the flowchart; we are just covering up—*suppressing*—bothersome symptoms. Rather than prescribing medication for everything, it would be better to concentrate on finding the root cause of the condition and try to reverse it. Understanding these general principles could help us prevent and treat everything from Alzheimer's and cancer, to opioid addiction and ADHD.

Now we also understand: combined together, the four immune-confusion disorders from above represent a *new class of archetypes* quietly sneaking into our lives—our new 21st century archetypes! The physical and emotional dysfunction on display, within those archetypes, is touching the core of what it means to be human, reminiscent of breaking the innermost center of a delicate machine. Yes, comparing the immune system, as a whole, to the central processing unit (CPU) of a computer might help us understand the amount of damage we have caused.

Planet Earth News

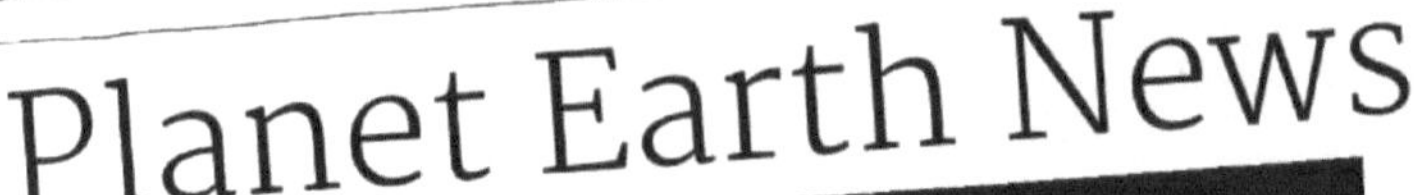

Mass Delusion At Immune System Army? First Attacking Bread, Then Each Other

****

Eyewitness Description:
"...there was blood everywhere..."

****

General Fairfite "Extremely Concerned" page 4

"...never seen anything like it..."
"...trust is gone..."

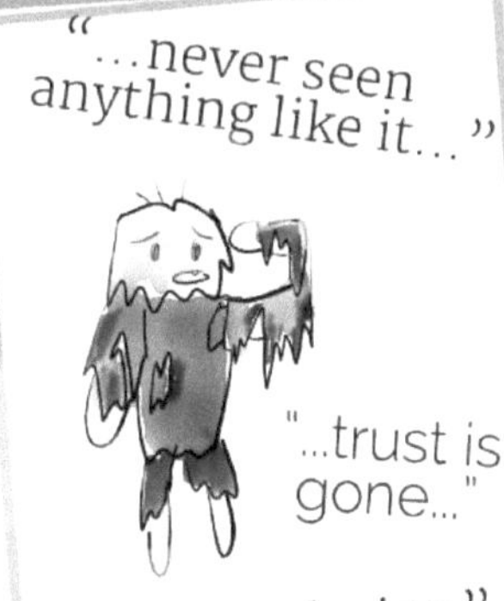

"total confusion"

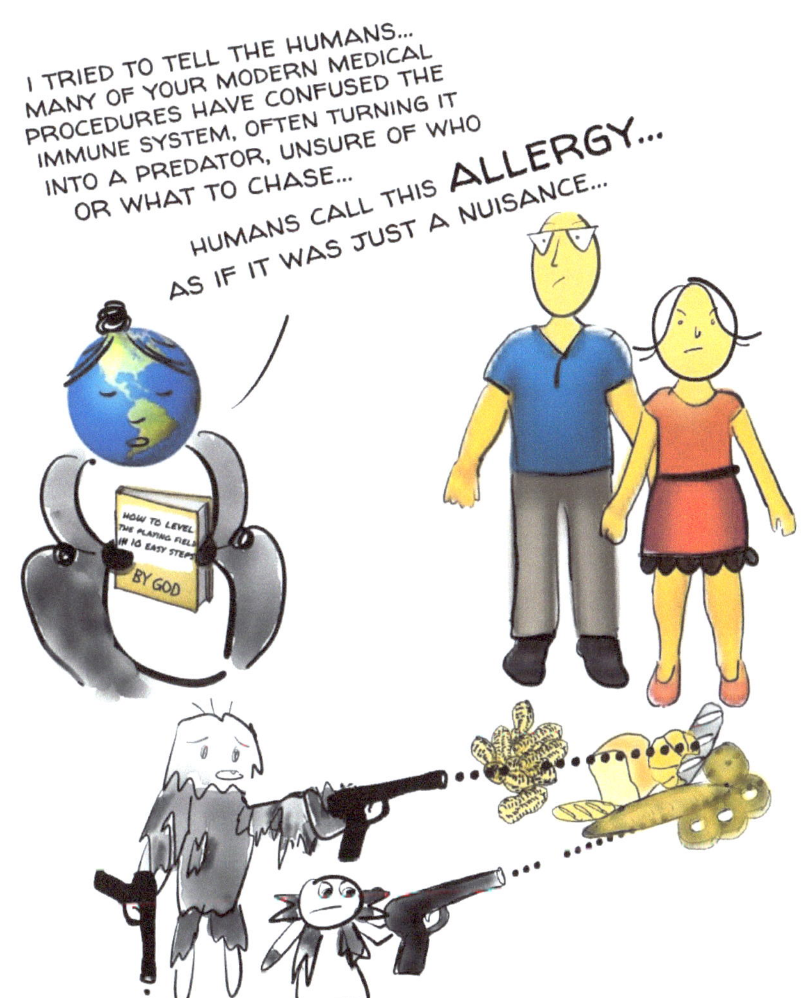
I TRIED TO TELL THE HUMANS...
MANY OF YOUR MODERN MEDICAL PROCEDURES HAVE CONFUSED THE IMMUNE SYSTEM, OFTEN TURNING IT INTO A PREDATOR, UNSURE OF WHO OR WHAT TO CHASE...
HUMANS CALL THIS ALLERGY...
AS IF IT WAS JUST A NUISANCE...
HOW TO LEVEL THE PLAYING FIELD IN 10 EASY STEPS
BY GOD

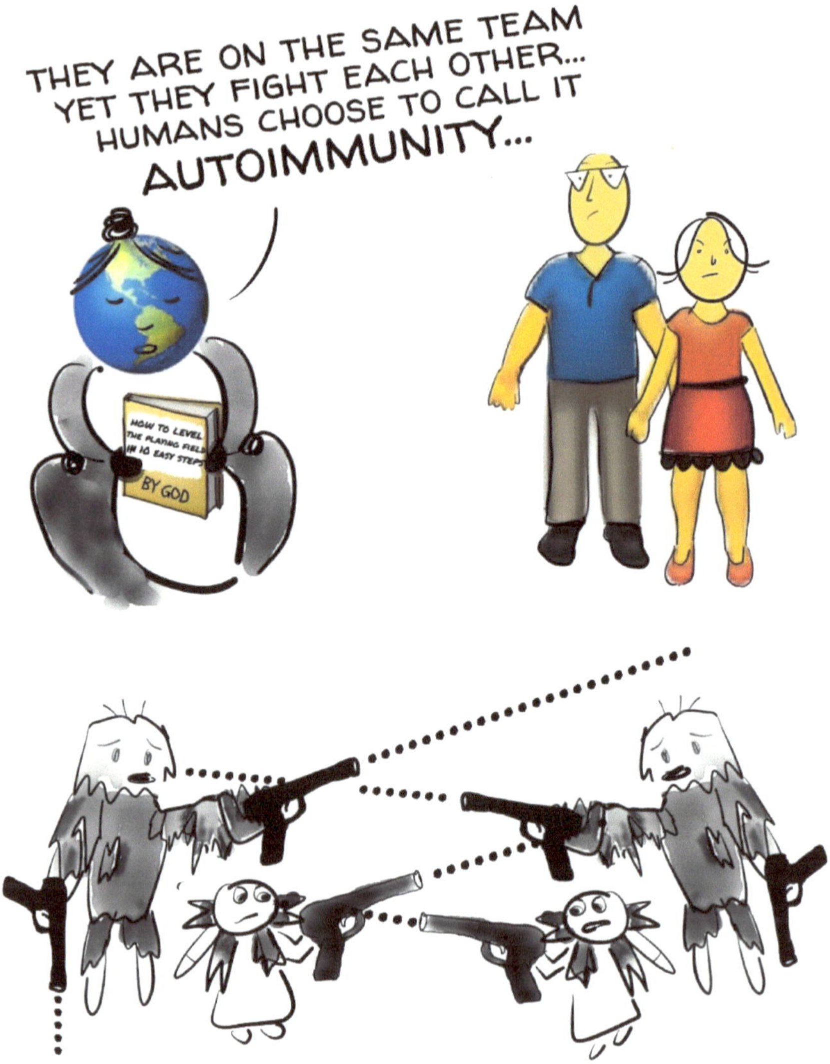

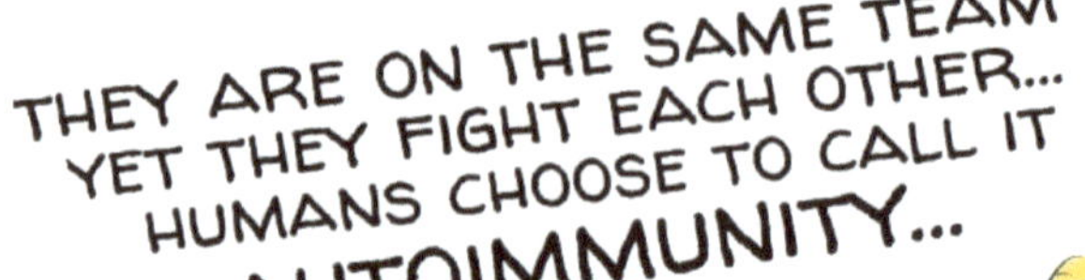

THEY ARE ON THE SAME TEAM
YET THEY FIGHT EACH OTHER...
HUMANS CHOOSE TO CALL IT
AUTOIMMUNITY...
HOW TO LEVEL
THE PLAYING FIELD
IN 10 EASY STEPS
BY GOD

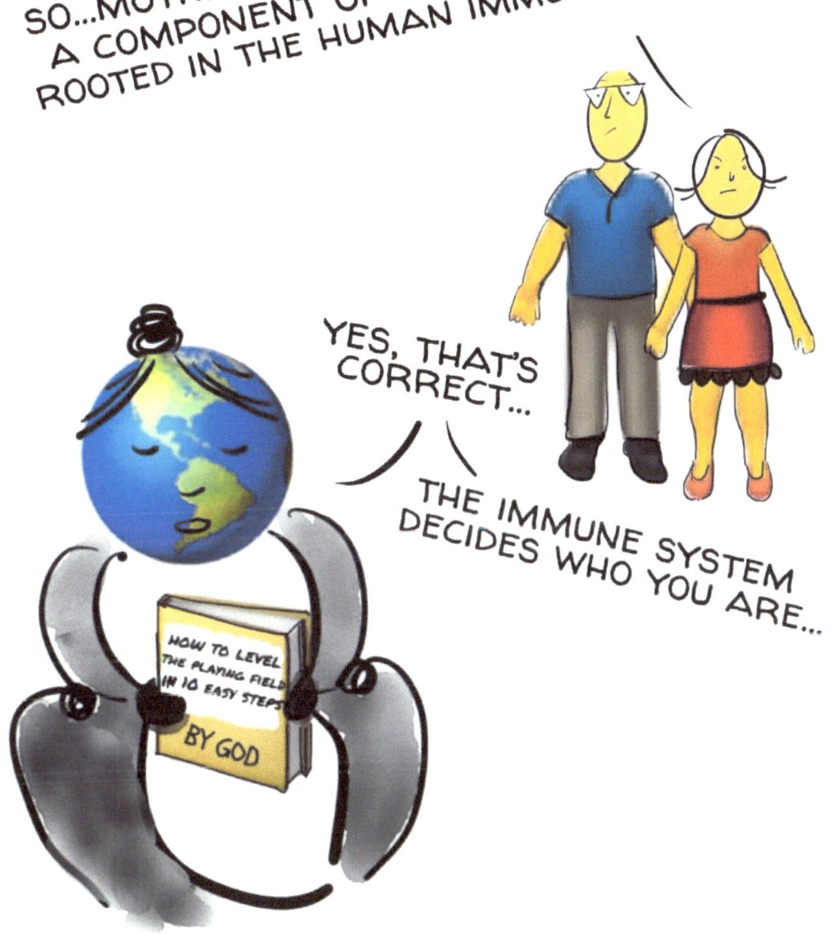
SO...MOTHER NATURE...THERE IS
A COMPONENT OF CONSCIOUSNESS
ROOTED IN THE HUMAN IMMUNE SYSTEM?
YES, THAT'S
CORRECT...
THE IMMUNE SYSTEM
DECIDES WHO YOU ARE...
HOW TO LEVEL
THE PLAYING FIELD
IN 10 EASY STEPS
BY GOD

Planet Earth News

"I want to destroy us!" Meaninglessness And Lack Of Challenge Give Rise To "Autoimmune Terrorism"
disturbing facts on page 7

What Is Consciousness?
An Interview With Staff From The Emotional And Mental Planes

The Central Question: Self and Non-Self page 10

Most Wanted

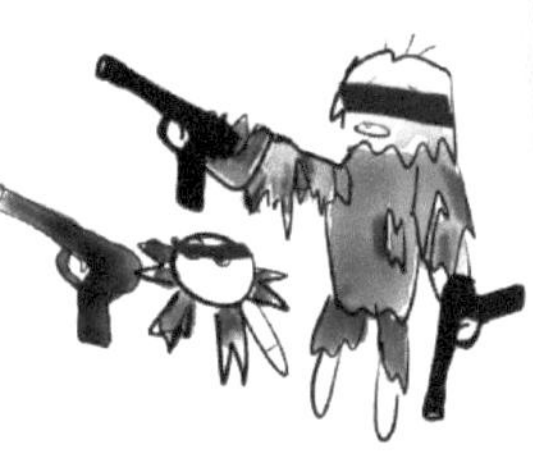

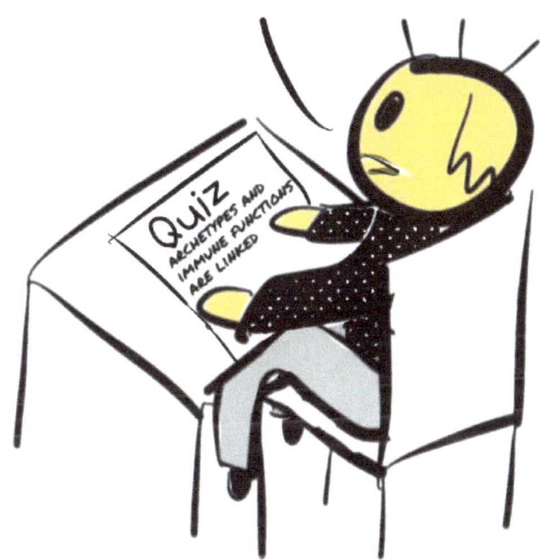
THIS QUIZ WAS NOT FUN!
IT WAS SCARY!
Quiz
ARCHETYPES AND
IMMUNE FUNCTIONS
ARE LINKED

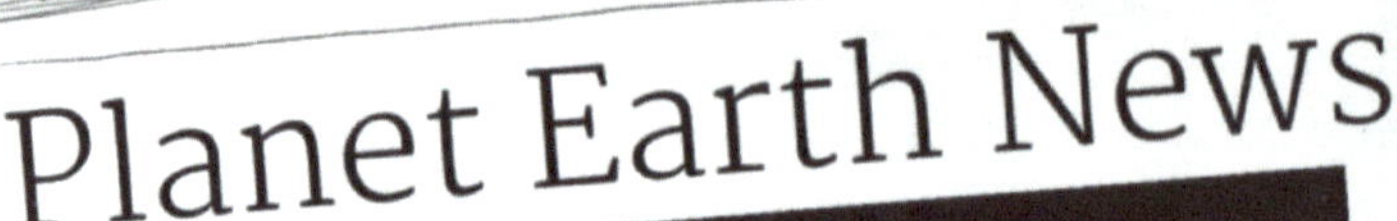

Planet Earth News

Immune System Training:
Stress in the Classroom

General Fairfite: Immune System Problems Systemic, Corruption Out Of Control! **page 10**

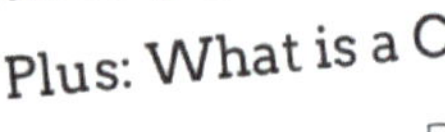

Plus: What is a CPU?

Students Stressed

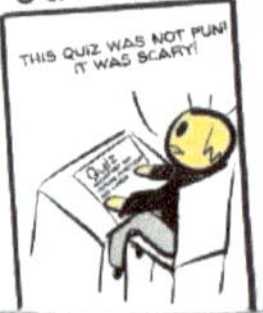

Immune System Dealing With New Disease Agents Never Seen Before: **"...strange and scary...like out of a sci-fi movie or a madman's lab..."**

go to page 5 for exclusive details

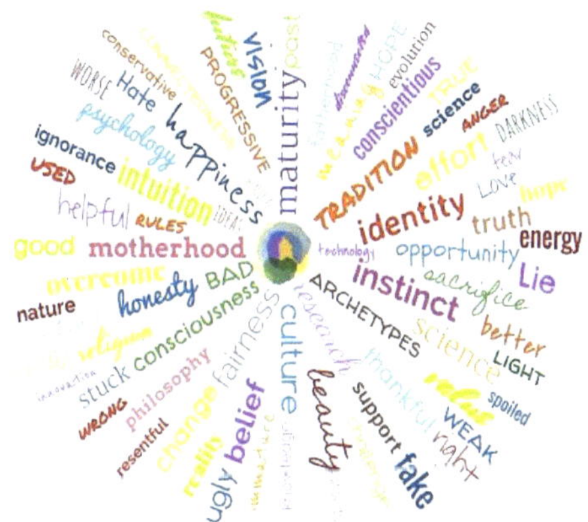
conservative
WORSE
Hate
psychology
happiness
ignorance
USED
intuition
helpful
RULES
IDEAS
good
motherhood
overcome
honesty
BAD
nature
religion
consciousness
stuck
philosophy
WRONG
fairness
change
resentful
reality
ugly
belief
culture
beauty
research
support
fake
thankful
right
WEAK
spoiled
LIGHT
science
better
ARCHETYPES
instinct
sacrifice
Lie
opportunity
energy
truth
identity
TRADITION
effort
Love
hope
DARKNESS
ANGER
science
conscientious
evolution
HOPE
maturity
past
vision
PROGRESSIVE
future

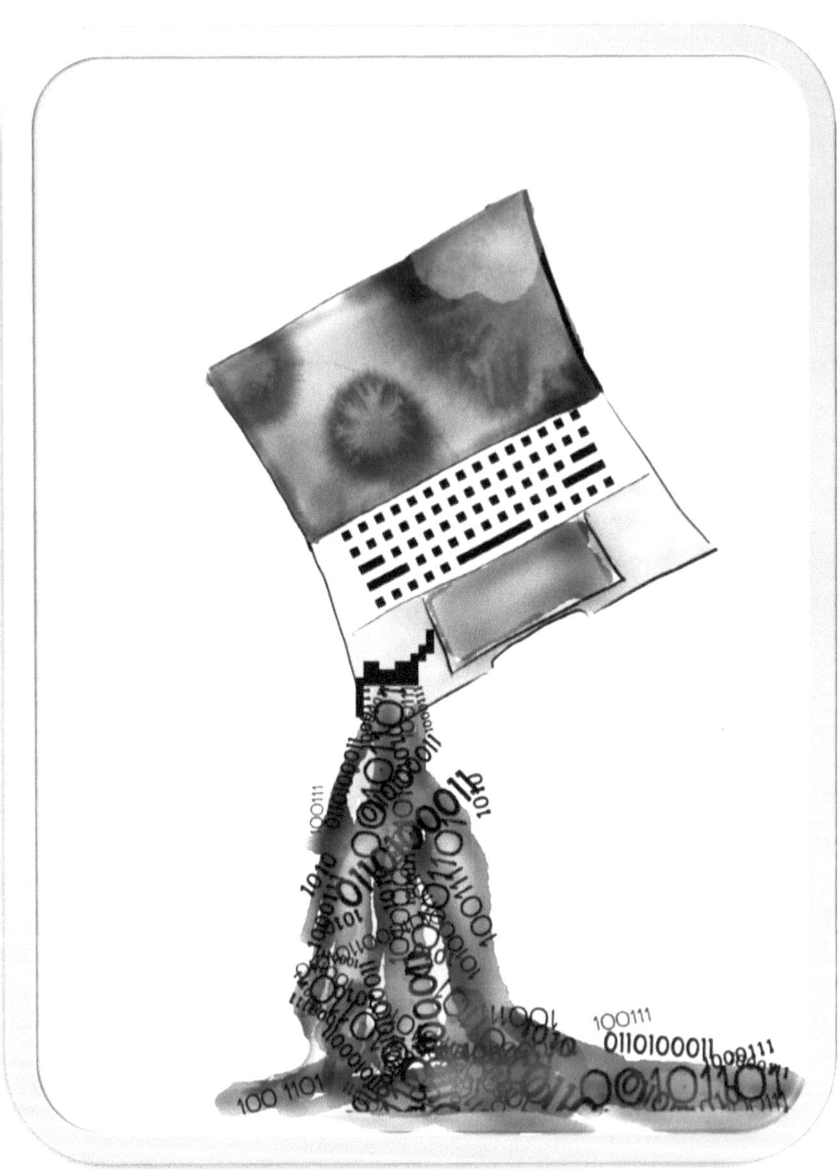
100111
100 1101

We Broke the CPU!

By Misna Burelli

Our immune system decides who we are, distinguishing between *self* and *non-self*, determining where we start and end, what is "us" and what is not "us". It makes judgements about friends versus enemies, implementing a complicated border control process, jailing all opponents of the system, while recognizing some visitors as harmless and granting them a temporary stay. There is a *hierarchy*: processes that *prioritize* some crucial sections of the body, like the head and heart, over other less important sections, like skin and intestines. This hierarchy helps to *preserve resources*, especially during emergencies. The whole system is geared towards *self-protection*, aiming for the best *long-term* outcome, not taking any chances. This beneficial kind of self-love is not too much—it's not automatically selfish but is able to see where sacrifice is necessary. There is no self-hate.

And here is what the immune system does not do: it does not let everyone in, especially not unchecked. It protects its own—what's precious—rather than playing around with "bad guys". It destroys them immediately or jails them. There is no taking false pity, but there is also no beating up innocent bystanders—it knows the difference. It is not unnecessarily aggressive, but then again it is also not politically correct. It does the right thing according to the golden rule. It is balanced...

Wait a minute...are you sure we are talking about the immune system? For a second, I was thinking we were talking about politics...

But actually, we are talking about politics! The emotional symptoms of the four *immune-confusion* diseases from above are reflected in current political discourse and society as a whole. This is the cultural emotional archetype that we currently live in, belonging to the new 21st century disease, called *Immune System Damage*. Our new miasm.

So why would immune system dysfunction—*damage*—as a whole, be reflected in today's societies? If you think about it, the immune system is really the innermost part of our being. It is our CPU. It determines who we are, what belongs to us—and what is outside of us.

Only the immune system knows. If you mix up those entities, you become someone else, or something else! Physical damage on that level would surely be reflected emotionally: it is destroying our essence, and our current culture shows it. Remember the three planes? Impairment shows on all three planes. The worse the harm, the more likely it will be displayed on the higher planes, such as the mental/emotional levels, forming a picture of the disease as a combination of all three planes.

This concept offers a reason for the millions of crisis conversations that seem to go nowhere, generating unworkable and impractical solutions, because in their naïveté, people simply claim that there are no problems. They can't see them—just like a damaged, unresponsive immune system, idly sitting around, watching its own destruction.

Or sometimes, it's the other way around: there is unexplainable hate and aggression toward innocent bystanders—people who have not done anything wrong are suddenly in the crossfire. It has been pointed out that today's society is exceedingly non-violent—unprecedented in human history.[59] Even though this observation is correct, it fails to consider a great deal of civilizing influence on modern day humans, separating them philosophically from their tribal ancestors. Today's kids are emotionally and intellectually far removed from any hunter-gatherer/warrior past and are explicitly taught to solve conflicts "with words". In contrast, our forefathers relied on strength, aggression, and physical power for their continued existence. The same is still true today for a number of tribal cultures around the world. The type of violence we see in these cultures often contributes to status, power, and sheer survival—an unnecessary element for most of us in the in the western world.

Instead, the current western expression of violence revolves around frustration, meaninglessness, oversensitivity, and general decay. ADHD, learning disabilities, lack of focus, anxiety attacks, and complete absence of energy are no assets. Constantly runny noses and itchy eyes get in the way of feeling well physically. For a lot of us, life has become

---

[59] Peterson, J.B. *12 Rules for Life: An Antidote to Chaos*, Random House Canada, **2018**, page 58

a drag, full of prescription medication, legal or illegal drugs, and special needs support—not a foundation for productive challenges. Self-hate and depression are at epidemic levels, confirming these concerns.[60] The effects of collectively disordered immune systems can be witnessed all around us: "emotional allergies", "emotional autoimmune diseases", and "emotional cancer" are everywhere on display; oversensitivity, aggression, lack of self-preservation skills, and a naïve type of immaturity are ubiquitous.

I'm not trying to paint an unnecessarily dark picture here—it is dark! It has become crucially important to turn this ship around, to heal the damage before we lose our ability to make rational decisions! The autism rate in children is already at a mind-boggling one in forty (2018)[61] —and worse in boys! What are we waiting for, and why is no one ringing the alarm? There are blogs, tracking the social and intellectual decay within our school systems, listing relevant news articles from mainstream media reports, and they are *scary*! Special needs budgets are out of control, teachers are suffering from burnout, cases of abuse of the disabled are skyrocketing, and too many additional counselors are needed just to run an ordinary school system.[62]

So many things already don't make sense: why do we constantly have to explain ourselves for wanting to protect ourselves and our loved ones? Why is it out of fashion to actually love ourselves and our loved ones with the kind of balanced self-love that is good for individuals, good for families, and good for society? Healthy self love, self-protection, and defense of our interests are not pathological at all—they are the foundation of a good society! People who have problems with self-love, doubting their own value, are often abused or become abusers themselves. They tend towards jealousy, a pattern of problematic relationships, constant anger and frustration, and the feeling of never having enough—not exactly a productive base for success!

---

[60] Miron, O. et al. Suicide Rates Among Adolescents and Young Adults in the United States, 2000-2017 *JAMA* **2019**; *321(23)*:2362-2364

[61] Kogan, M.D. The Prevalence of Parent-Reported Autism Spectrum Disorder Among US Children, *Pediatrics*, **2018,** *142(6),* 1-11

[62] Lossofbraintrust.com

Other times, we are accused of discrimination when not cheerfully including everyone, even the bullies. We are reminded that we are not allowed to openly dislike others, no matter the circumstances. Whole inclusion departments have sprung up in our schools, fully ignoring the fact that standards are necessary for inclusion to be successful. On the other hand, at the transition to university, almost everyone is excluded; benchmarks—based mostly on a résumé of busywork in combination with identity politics—are impossible to reach for most. In addition, an ever-growing percentage of "elite disabled" are now admitted to famous colleges—perhaps as many as one in four.[63] No one in charge seems to be remotely concerned about any resentment arising from giving these students extra time on tests, while many "non-disabled" are not even admitted.

We are often prompted to make huge sacrifices for unknown causes, solving short-term problems with unclear long-term goals and outcomes because this is "who we are". And there you have it: in the new age of immune system confusion, we actually have no idea who we are, what we stand for, what values we should defend, and even what direction we should take in life—we just follow simple recipes, feeling good about ourselves rather than producing results. We are so involved with ourselves that there is no room for answering the larger questions of life—focusing on greater principles and higher ideals—while doubting even the most basic elements of humanity. Having lost our intuition and instincts, we seem to be obsessed with all kinds of identity issues, constantly trying to find our true selves and even switching identities, if we feel in any way mismatched.

There are many current social trends which have to do with immune dysfunction, and transgender issues are among them. If you don't know yourself on the emotional level, how do you know if you are male or female? Just looking at those parts is not enough, there has to be agreement throughout the whole body, on all planes! But if the emotional immune system—on the second plane—declines to do the

---

63 Colleges Bend the Rules for More Students, Give Them Extra Help, *The Wall Street Journal*, May 24, **2018**

final quality control check, refusing to confirm your sex on an emotional level, you can't be sure if those parts are right. So you feel off. It's simply an emotional response to an open question—the body is constantly trying to find the self. It is a mismatch on the plane levels. Homeopaths tend to call this an incarnation problem, but that's just fancy speak for the fact that the mental/emotional body and the physical body don't align correctly. This also relates to the "feminine chaos" versus "masculine order" archetype theory mentioned earlier; male and female immune system archetypes display noticeable differences, expressing themselves as gender dependent in terms of rates of ADHD, autism, anxiety, and depression.

And by the way, this is *not* an endorsement to harass transsexuals or other groups that appear to be suffering from the immune dysfunction miasm. Instead, it is an attempt to explain what is happening, allowing everyone to make their own, albeit more informed, decisions. It is certainly complicated and involves real pain and suffering. Therefore, I can't overemphasize how important it is for us to be able to express ourselves freely, creating an environment where opposing views are allowed to flourish and incorporating both poles into our discussions. Only then will it be possible to find true lasting solutions—through *balance.*

There have been cases of similar feelings of mismatch arising regarding other body parts, like arms and legs, leading people to insist on wanting to amputate the "wrong parts". But it is the same thing: the immune system got confused, forgetting to check off the physical parts and the emotional body as belonging together, and now the body is puzzled that it can't find them on all three planes, leading to the decision that they must be wrong.

Since all of the above identity concerns have their roots in immune system dysfunction, finding the real self is a matter of healing on all three levels (*physical, mental and emotional*) and putting the three planes back together the way they were meant to be. This is no small task, but well worth the effort, since, according to Jung, "the privilege of a lifetime is to become who you truly are". While I completely agree with this statement, it needs to be pointed out that he was probably not aware of the great impact of health on this emotional goal.

I would also like to add that finding the real you is never a forced procedure; instead, it happens in a natural way by clearing up confusion. Clearing up confusion is preferred, as it will make people feel healthier and happier overall. Our bodies work best when we are strong on all three planes, and all planes agree with each other. This is a tall order, and most of us won't qualify fully, but it is clearly the best prerequisite for finding the true you, and for all planes to come together properly. Starting slowly, every little bit of improvement makes us feel better, and even if we don't reach this destination completely, we can, and should try. No one has to be perfect!

And the preferred way to get there? By improving the immune system!

Yes, you can just start with this first simple step: dealing with the immune system specific archetype picture—on all planes, of course—overlapping with your inborn, natural archetype. Once the immune system confusion lifts, many things will change for the better, and it will become possible to discover and heal the true you!

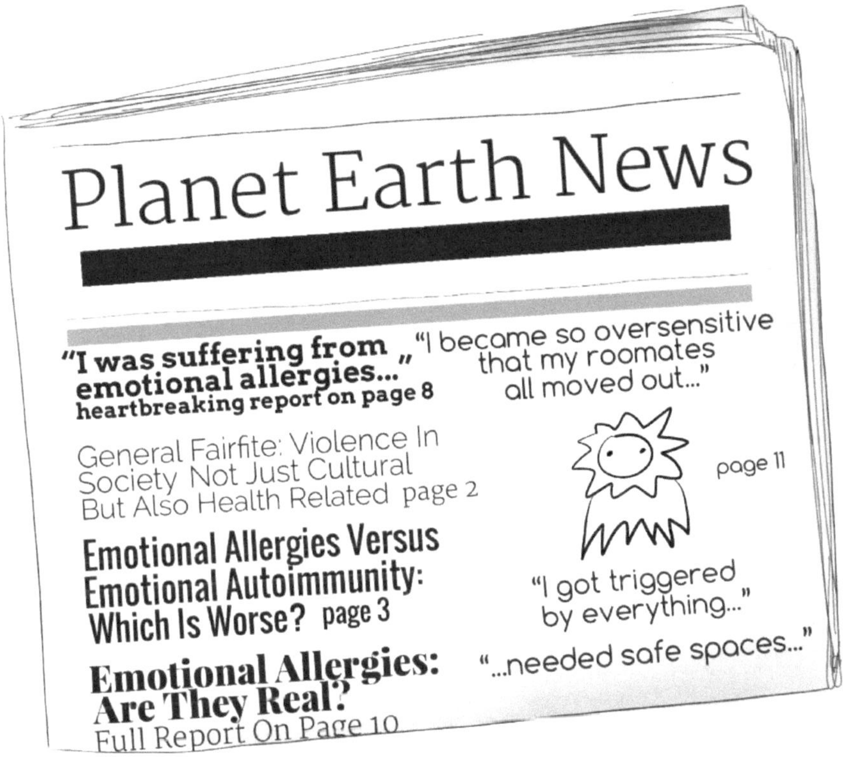

Planet Earth News

"I was suffering from emotional allergies..."
heartbreaking report on page 8

"I became so oversensitive that my roomates all moved out..."

General Fairfite: Violence In Society Not Just Cultural But Also Health Related page 2

page 11

Emotional Allergies Versus Emotional Autoimmunity: Which Is Worse? page 3

"I got triggered by everything..."

"...needed safe spaces..."

Emotional Allergies: Are They Real?
Full Report On Page 10

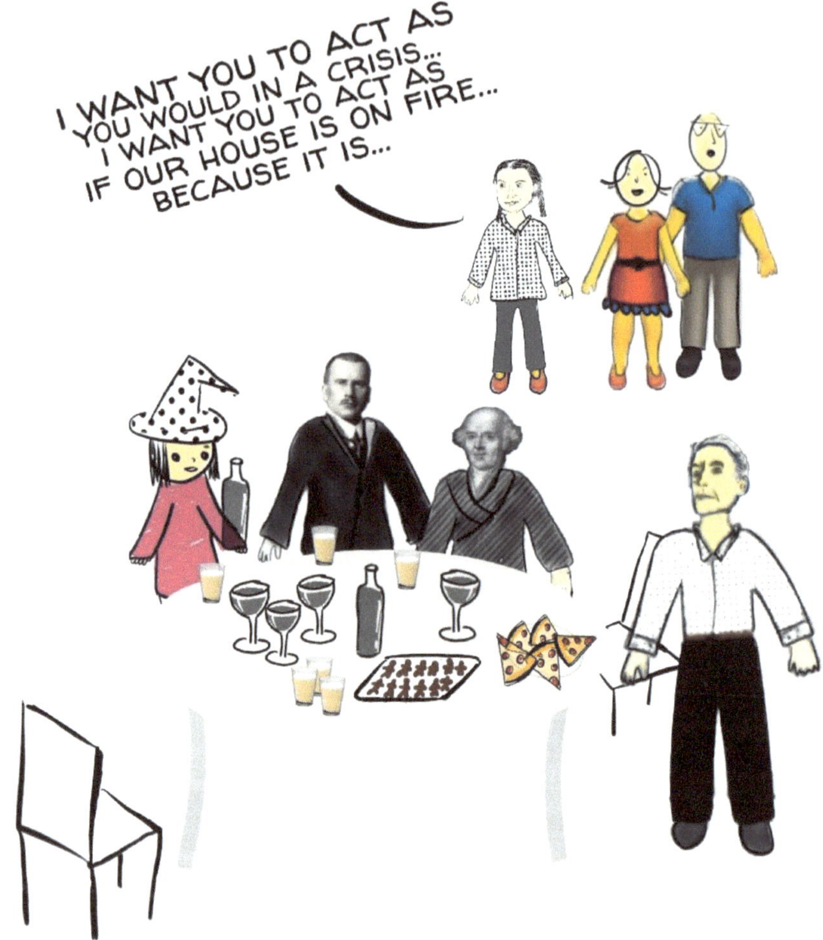
I WANT YOU TO ACT AS
YOU WOULD IN A CRISIS...
I WANT YOU TO ACT AS
IF OUR HOUSE IS ON FIRE...
BECAUSE IT IS...

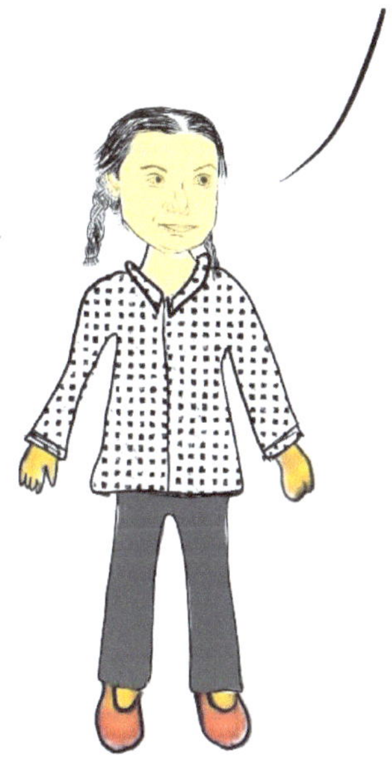
OUR CIVILIZATION IS BEING SACRIFICED FOR THE OPPORTUNITY OF A VERY SMALL NUMBER OF PEOPLE TO CONTINUE MAKING ENORMOUS AMOUNTS OF MONEY...

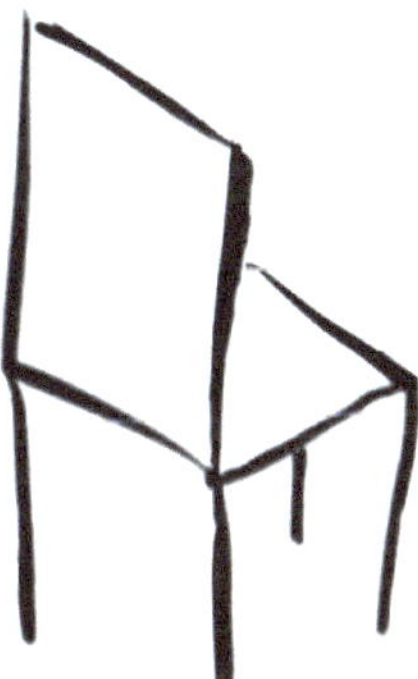

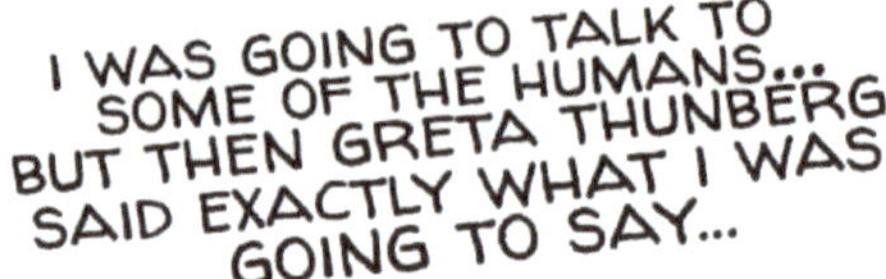
I WAS GOING TO TALK TO
SOME OF THE HUMANS...
BUT THEN GRETA THUNBERG
SAID EXACTLY WHAT I WAS
GOING TO SAY...

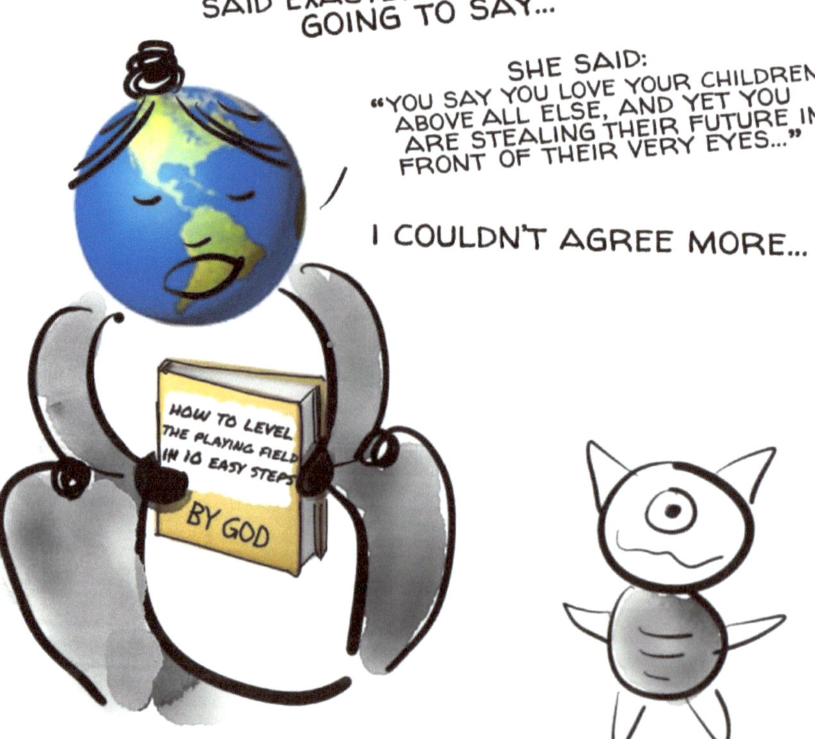
SHE SAID:
"YOU SAY YOU LOVE YOUR CHILDREN ABOVE ALL ELSE, AND YET YOU ARE STEALING THEIR FUTURE IN FRONT OF THEIR VERY EYES..."
I COULDN'T AGREE MORE...
HOW TO LEVEL THE PLAYING FIELD IN 10 EASY STEPS
BY GOD

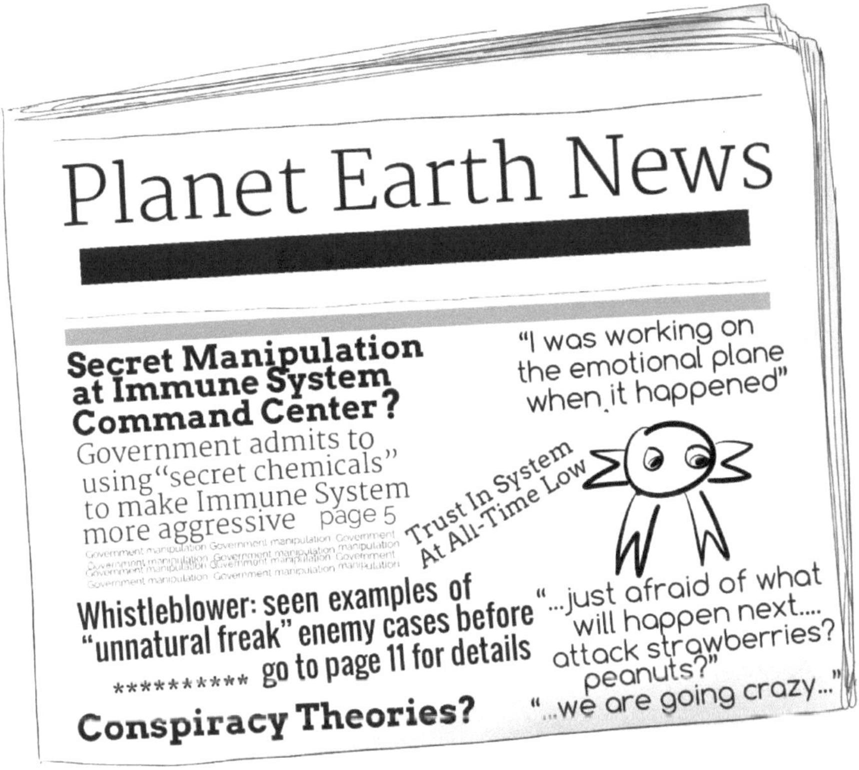

Planet Earth News

Secret Manipulation at Immune System Command Center?

Government admits to using "secret chemicals" to make Immune System more aggressive page 5

"I was working on the emotional plane when it happened"

Trust In System At All-Time Low

Whistleblower: seen examples of "unnatural freak" enemy cases before go to page 11 for details

"...just afraid of what will happen next.... attack strawberries? peanuts?"

****

Conspiracy Theories?

"...we are going crazy..."

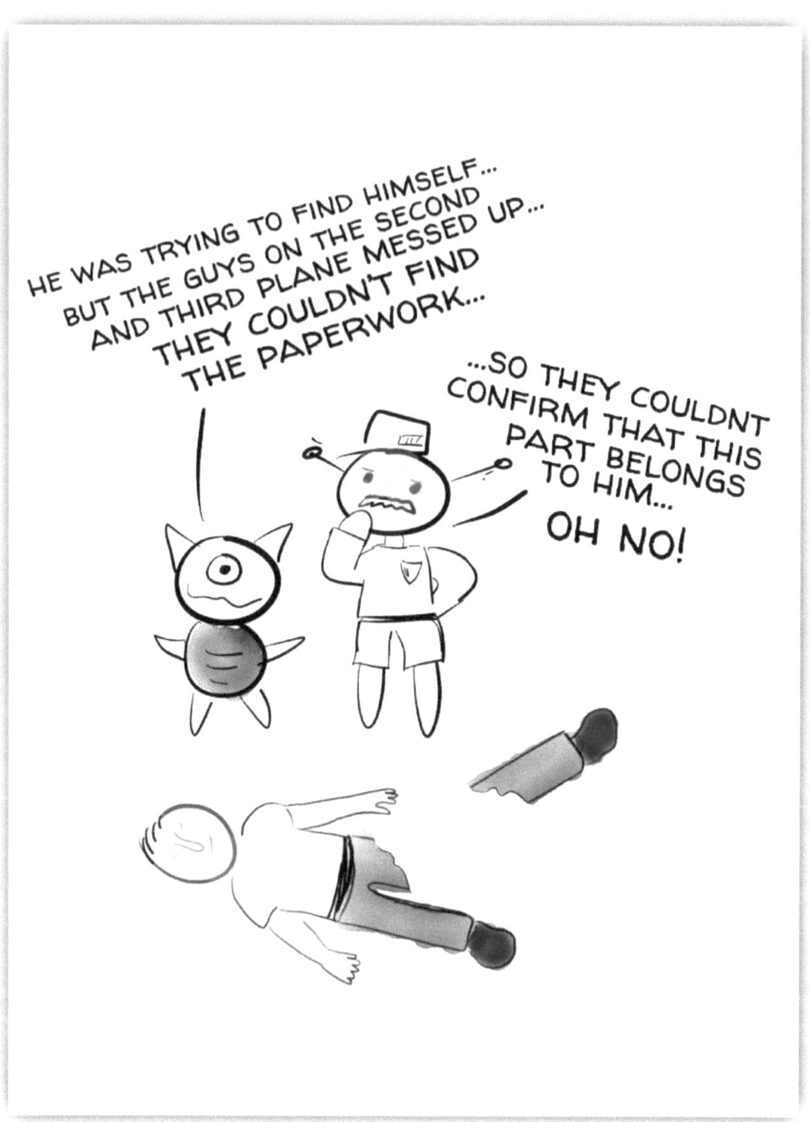
HE WAS TRYING TO FIND HIMSELF...
BUT THE GUYS ON THE SECOND
AND THIRD PLANE MESSED UP...
THEY COULDN'T FIND
THE PAPERWORK...
...SO THEY COULDNT
CONFIRM THAT THIS
PART BELONGS
TO HIM...
OH NO!

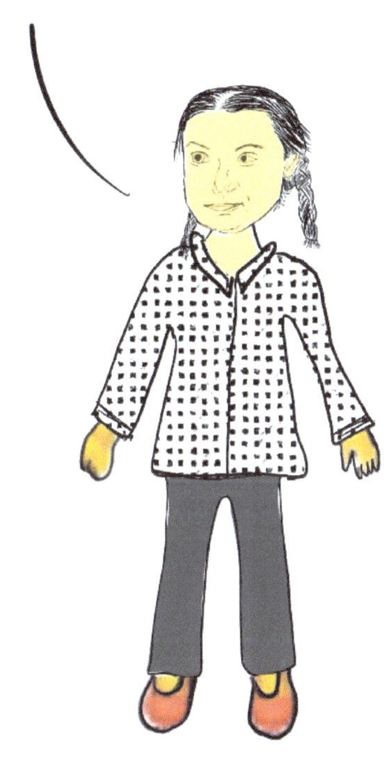
YOU SAY YOU LOVE YOUR CHILDREN ABOVE ALL ELSE, AND YET YOU ARE STEALING THEIR FUTURE IN FRONT OF THEIR VERY EYES...

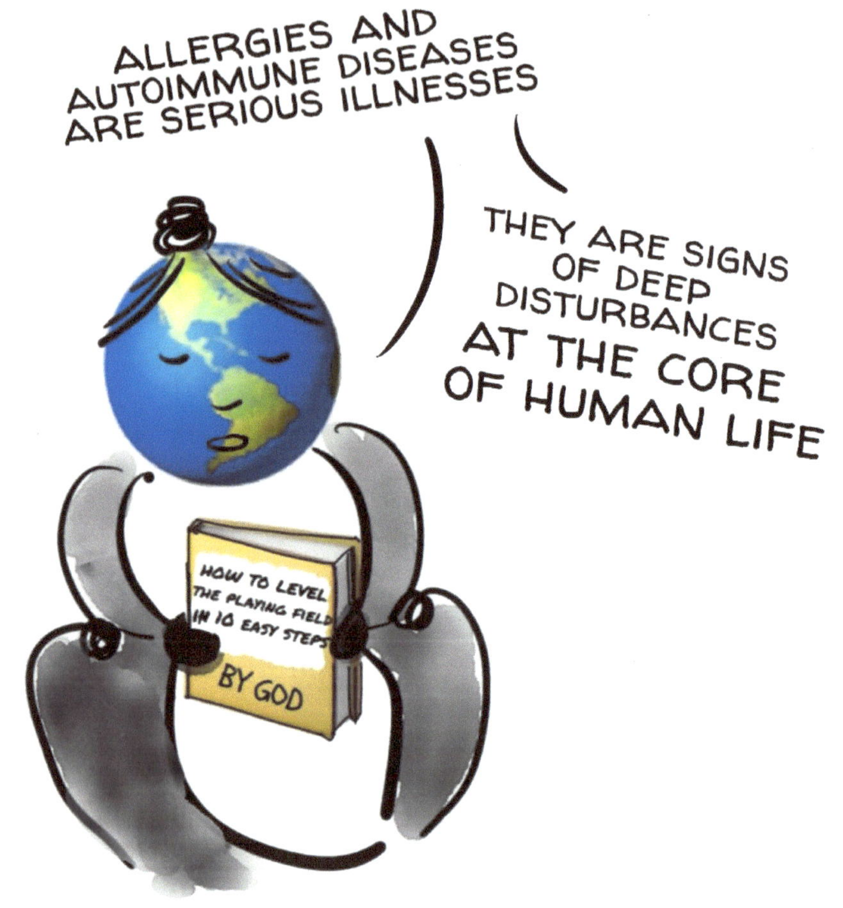
ALLERGIES AND AUTOIMMUNE DISEASES ARE SERIOUS ILLNESSES
THEY ARE SIGNS OF DEEP DISTURBANCES AT THE CORE OF HUMAN LIFE
HOW TO LEVEL THE PLAYING FIELD IN 10 EASY STEPS
BY GOD

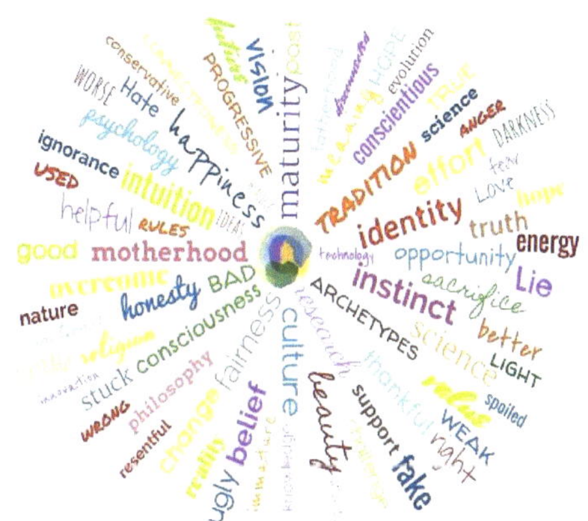
maturity
vision
PROGRESSIVE
conservative
WORSE
Hate
psychology
happiness
ignorance
USED
intuition
helpful
RULES
IDEAS
good
motherhood
honesty
BAD
nature
consciousness
stuck
philosophy
WRONG
resentful
change
fairness
ugly
belief
culture
beauty
support
fake
thankful
right
WEAK
spoiled
LIGHT
better
science
ARCHETYPES
instinct
sacrifice
Lie
opportunity
energy
truth
identity
technology
TRADITION
effort
LOVE
DARKNESS
ANGER
science
conscientious
evolution

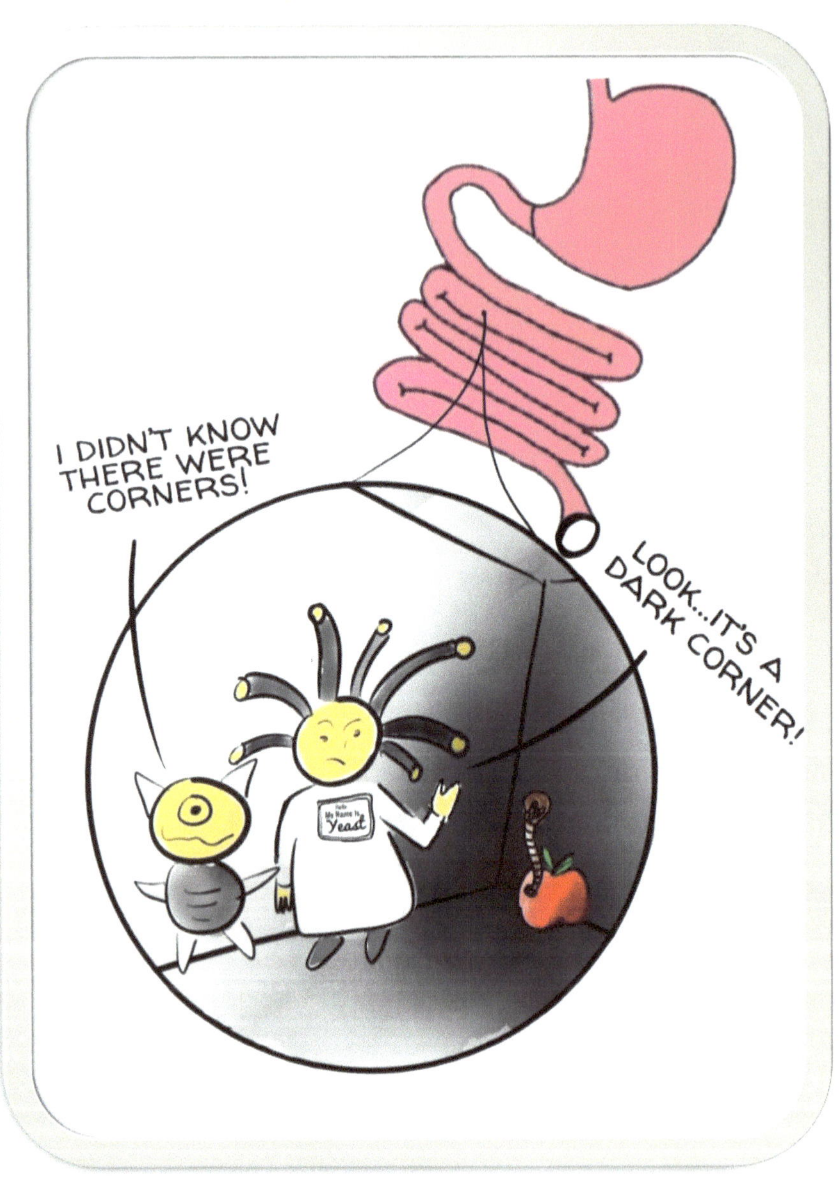
I DIDN'T KNOW THERE WERE CORNERS!
LOOK...IT'S A DARK CORNER!
My Name Is
Yeast

Back to the Dark Corners of the Gut

By Lena Kratz

Let's make a plan: we would like to improve our health by re-tuning our immune system. Great—but how do we get started? As explained in the last chapter, most diseases are rooted in immune system dysfunction, even mental/emotional ones.

One of the first things we can do is to stop using suppressive medications/procedures as our go-to choices of medical care. The body creates symptoms, even uncomfortable ones, for a reason. Not allowing the body to express itself leads to the disorder being pushed deeper onto the second and third planes. Recovery is a reversal process: bringing symptoms back from the second and third planes—the emotional and mental ones—to the first plane. It has been noticed that in more serious cases of illness, the body is often unable to express itself at all on the first plane—the physical one. Autistic children or Alzheimer's patients often display mostly second and third plane pathologies rather than physical symptoms—no colds, fevers, and runny noses. This often confuses caretakers into thinking that their child or parent is "very healthy"—except for the mental/emotional disorder. It is the opposite: they are so ill that they are unable to express physical symptoms. We can tell that recovery is setting in when illness comes back to the physical plane: we develop a sore throat, a rash, or a fever, replacing some of the mental/emotional symptoms. This immune system boost is a sure sign that we are on the right path!

In addition to avoiding suppression, we can take a number of steps to proactively encourage our immune systems to regenerate themselves. Many people have had success concerning this matter, addressing a variety of health conditions. So, let's take a look at their health recovery stories. Analyzing them for a common thread, with the goal of engineering a plan out of those bits and pieces, will give us a starting point. An abundance of such stories can be found around autism.[64] This is probably due to the fact that mainstream medical facilities often have nothing to offer autistic patients and their parents; failing to provide effective treatment options, parents seek out their own paths.[65]

Among a multitude of therapies,[66] [67] including what is called the biomedical approach to autism,[68] a definite common thread for recovery is diet:[69] people usually start with organic, often switching to gluten free, then low carb or SCD (specific carbohydrate diet) and ending up with paleo or even only meat. It makes sense that there is a connection to the immune system—many scientists have pointed out the links between gut flora and certain foods, highlighting how the bacterial makeup inside the intestines can be altered through diet and probiotics.[70] After all, a large part of our immune system—perhaps up to 70%, in what is called the gut associated lymphatic tissue or GALT— resides in the gut.

There is no one-size-fits-all: diet changes work better for some people than for others, depending on the severity of the damage, the type of probiotic, intestinal infections, levels of stomach acid, allergies etc. But overall, success has been documented, and support groups of all kinds have sprung up all over the country.[71]

There is only one thing missing: changing the bacterial gut flora often doesn't adequately address fungal or parasite infections. Even the best epidemiologists are completely in the dark about this, claiming that no one in the developed western world would ever suffer from intestinal

---

[64] Whiffen, L. *A Child's Journey Out of Autism: One Family's Story of Living in Hope and Finding a Cure*, Sourcebooks, Inc. Naperville, Illinois, **2009**
[65] Bock, K. *Healing the New Childhood Epidemics: Autism, ADHD, Asthma and Allergies* Ballantine Books, New York, **2008**
[66] Herbert, M. and Weintraub, K. *The Autism Revolution: whole-body strategies for making life all it can be*, Ballantine Books, **2013**
[67] Jepson, B. *Changing the Course of Autism: A Scientific Approach for Parents and Physicians*, Sentient Publications, **2007**
[68] Edelson, S.M. and Rimland, B. *Recovering Autistic Children*, Autism Research Institute, **2006**
[69] Baker, S. and Pangborn, J. *Autism: Have We Done Everything We Can for This Child? Effective Biomedical Treatments*, Autism Research Institute, **2005**
[70] Gottschall, E. *Breaking The Vicious Cycle: Intestinal Health through Diet*, Kirkton Press Ltd, **1994**
[71] westonaprice.org

worms.

Homeopaths naturally disagree. How can we tell? Lets' get to this in a minute. Let me ask you a question first: have you ever taken an antiparasitic medication? *Yes?* Did you know that this conventional treatment is best started according to lunar phases?

I'm not joking—it is a well-known fact that antiparasitic medications are more effective when taken according to the moon cycle. Drug manufacturers are aware of this, even if doctors usually don't mention it.[72] Mebendazole, one of the main anti-parasitic drugs, has been in the news as a re-purposed medication for cancer.[73] Surprised scientists have been scrambling to come up with a mechanism of action[74]—but could it possibly be the parasites themselves that tip a weak immune system into cancer? There are enough suspicious connections between parasites and cancer that this hypothesis doesn't seem too far-fetched. We will discuss some of these connections later in another chapter.

But homeopaths have another way to know—by looking at the remedy pictures! Many emotional archetypes include sensitivity to the moon cycle, which is an indication for parasite infection. *Yes, I know what you are thinking!* There are many articles, usually citing anecdotal evidence only, which speculate on the connections between hospital emergency visits and full moons. Or we could just ask teachers: a few years ago, a second-grade teacher we know admitted that—in her opinion—the moon cycle plays a major role in children's behavior, causing them to act out on days during the full moon. According to her it was undeniable, taking place every month, making the classroom environment more difficult. Even though it was meant to be a funny anecdote at the time, it left no room for arguments.

But why would the full moon lead to moon behavior? Very

---

72 Dr. Schmidt's blog at The Nutritional Healing Center of Ann Arbor at thenutritionalhealingcenter.com

73 Pantsiarka, P. et al. Repurposing Drugs in Oncology (ReDO)-mebendazole as an anti-cancer agent *Ecancermedicalscience* **2014**, *8*: 443

74 Guerini, A. E. et al. Mebendazole as a Candidate for Drug Repurposing in Oncology: An Extensive Review of Current Literature *Cancers (Basel)*, **2019**, *11*(9):1284

simple: worm's reproductive cycles orient themselves by the moon, producing behavioral symptoms through their activities and the release of toxins during that time.

So, all of this points toward the uncomfortable truth that we humans might frequently harbor parasites. Some of the most worm prone archetypal pictures are common remedies such as *silica* (sand), *cina* (wormseed), *teucrium*, and *nat phos. Cina,* especially, is a remedy which does not only treat worm infestations but also tension, anxiety, and sleeping difficulties. In fact, the FDA regulated homoeopathic pharmacopeia of the United States (HPUS) asks homeopathic manufacturers to list several symptoms that are associated with the remedies, and for *cina* this includes: nervousness, irritability, and sleeplessness in children—are these symptoms directly connected to parasites?

The idea that we could all be suffering from worm infestations was a major revelation for me at the time, because it turns out that worms are *really bad* for you, playing a major factor in many chronic disease processes. This includes anxiety, obesity, autism, OCD, brain fog, mood swings, insomnia—parasites are active at night—liver problems and, as just mentioned, possibly even cancer. Perhaps they affect brain function directly. If Kathleen McAuliffe's book titled *This is Your Brain on Parasites: How Tiny Creatures Manipulate our Behavior and Shape Society* is any indication, we should probably start worrying right now.[75] Stories about parasite-infected "hijacked suicidal zombie" snails or fish launching themselves right into the arms of their predators have raised eyebrows among biologists—could similar behavior manipulation happen to human hosts?[76]

Unfortunately, worms are extremely difficult to get rid of. Since we all seem to host at least a few of them, any dip in the immune system can be detrimental, giving them an opportunity to increase their

---

[75] McAuliffe, K. *This is Your Brain on Parasites: How Tiny Creatures Manipulate our Behavior and Shape Society* Eamon Dolan/Mariner Books, **2017**

[76] Swartz, S. J et al. Infection with schistosome parasites in snails leads to increased predation by pawns: implications for human schistosomiasis control *Journal of Experimental Biology* **2015**, *218*, 3962-3967

territory. Many cultures around the world are intuitively aware of these dangers, preventing the spread of parasites with herbs and hot spices. Nature has equipped us with additional mechanisms to avoid exposure: strong feelings of disgust signal us to stay away from filthy, slimy trash or unsanitary living conditions. This healthy reaction is simply a self-protective mechanism, preventing parasites from gaining the upper hand.

There are some autism parents who think that parasites—in combination with a chronically weak immune system—are at the root of the disease. They have a point: autistic symptoms can start suddenly, without warning—might there be a link to an unfortunate lapse in immune system function, giving parasites an advantage to take over a weakened body? These same autism parents have also published an autism recovery protocol based on the elimination of worms; viewing the results in the toilet can be disturbing—sometimes the creatures can exceed thirty-nine inches!

A number of children have recovered or dramatically improved after following this protocol, which is based on a number of treatments, including the anthelmintic drugs pyrantel pamoate and mebendazole. Details of their recovery stories have been documented in the book *Healing the Symptoms known as Autism.*[77]

Reading through some of the recovery accounts, it is interesting to note that, just like in homeopathy, true healing stories often include a "return of old symptoms" —the body produces symptoms that were seen a while ago and then forgotten. It appears to be a hallmark of true cures. We will discuss "return of old symptoms" later in another chapter.

To summarize: the above shows that a combination of diet and medication—or even fecal transplants[78]—can often work wonders, improving a broken immune system even in situations that might seem almost hopeless otherwise. And, of course, I would add homeopathy to the mix.

So, what happens when people really do get better, healing their intestines and losing their diagnosis? They improve on every level:

[77] Rivera, K. *Healing the Symptoms Known as Autism*, **2014**
[78] Mikhaila Peterson at mikhailapeterson.com

physically, emotionally and mentally. On the physical plane, stomach and intestinal pains are perhaps lessened or disappear completely; on the emotional plane the oversensitivity and anxiety vanish; and on the mental plane, the ADHD is fading away. There is progress everywhere: academically, emotionally, and socially.

Sometimes newly recovered individuals will even say: "I think my friend is actually not a good friend…I suddenly see this now. I don't like her anymore. I don't know why I haven't seen this before…but I think she's mean, and she was using me. I can't let this happen again".

With a newly functioning immune system and improved emotional borders in place, bullying or other school-related social concerns often vanish like snow in the sun, and peace comes back to the family. For older people, the same often happens in the workplace—they become more comfortable in their skin, easily handling everyday obstacles and stress. Family members are frequently surprised by such a personality change, but, in reality, it is no change at all: it is personality damage that got repaired. Healing physical symptoms often leads to a newly found assertiveness and a desire to stand up for one's balanced values. Individuals are finally finding themselves, taking their rightful place in society. They are ready to become who they truly are.

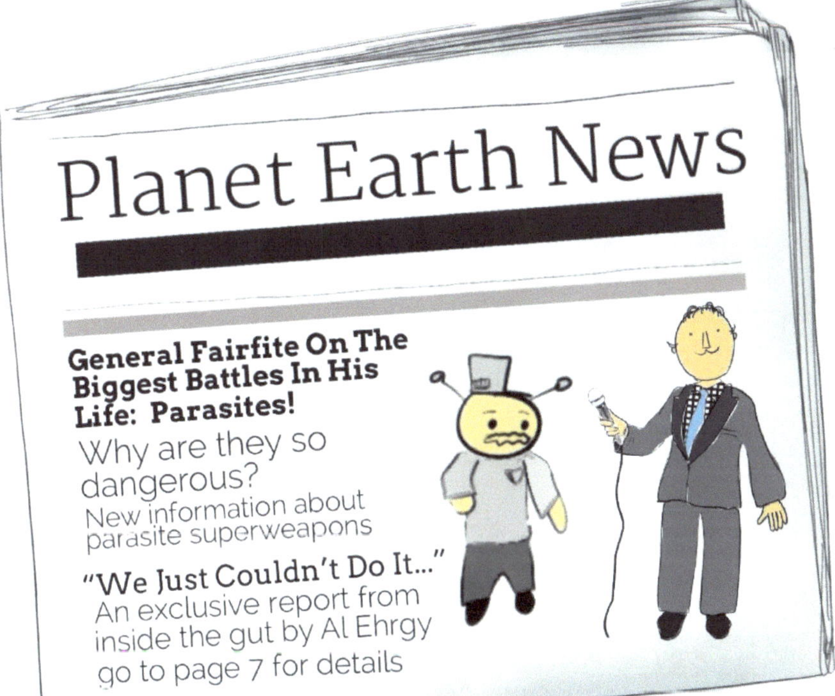
Planet Earth News

General Fairfite On The Biggest Battles In His Life: Parasites!

Why are they so dangerous?

New information about parasite superweapons

"We Just Couldn't Do It..."

An exclusive report from inside the gut by Al Ehrgy

go to page 7 for details

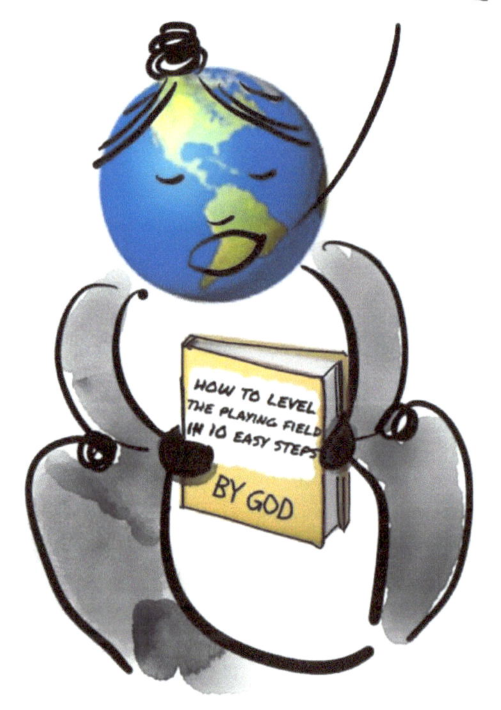
MATURITY HAPPENS WHEN WE TRAIN THE IMMUNE SYSTEM...
HOW TO LEVEL THE PLAYING FIELD IN 10 EASY STEPS
BY GOD

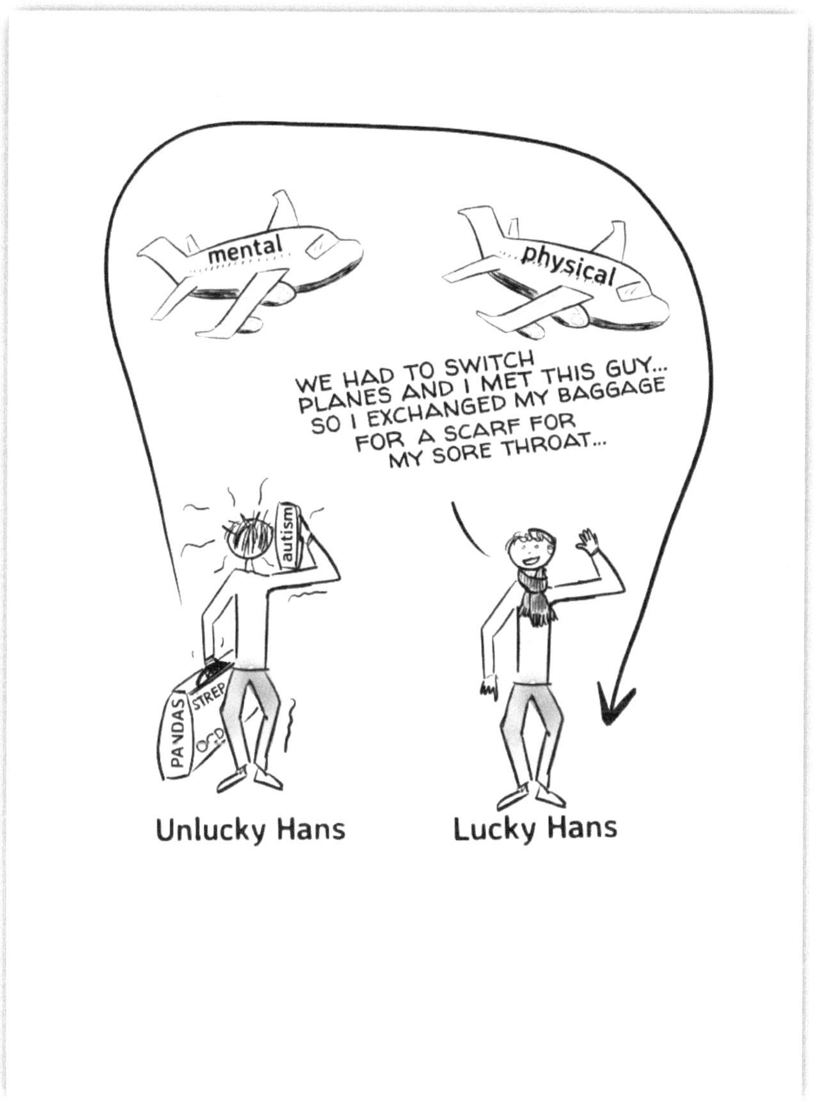

Homeopathic Fairy Tales:
Hans in Luck

THERE IS ONLY GOODNESS OUT THERE...THIS APPLE LOOKS JUICY... WHAT A NICE LADY... COMING FROM SO FAR AWAY... JUST TO GIVE ME AN APPLE...
PRINCESS! DANGER!! DON'T YOU SEE IT?
I LOVE STRINGS... WAIT...IT'S A WORM!

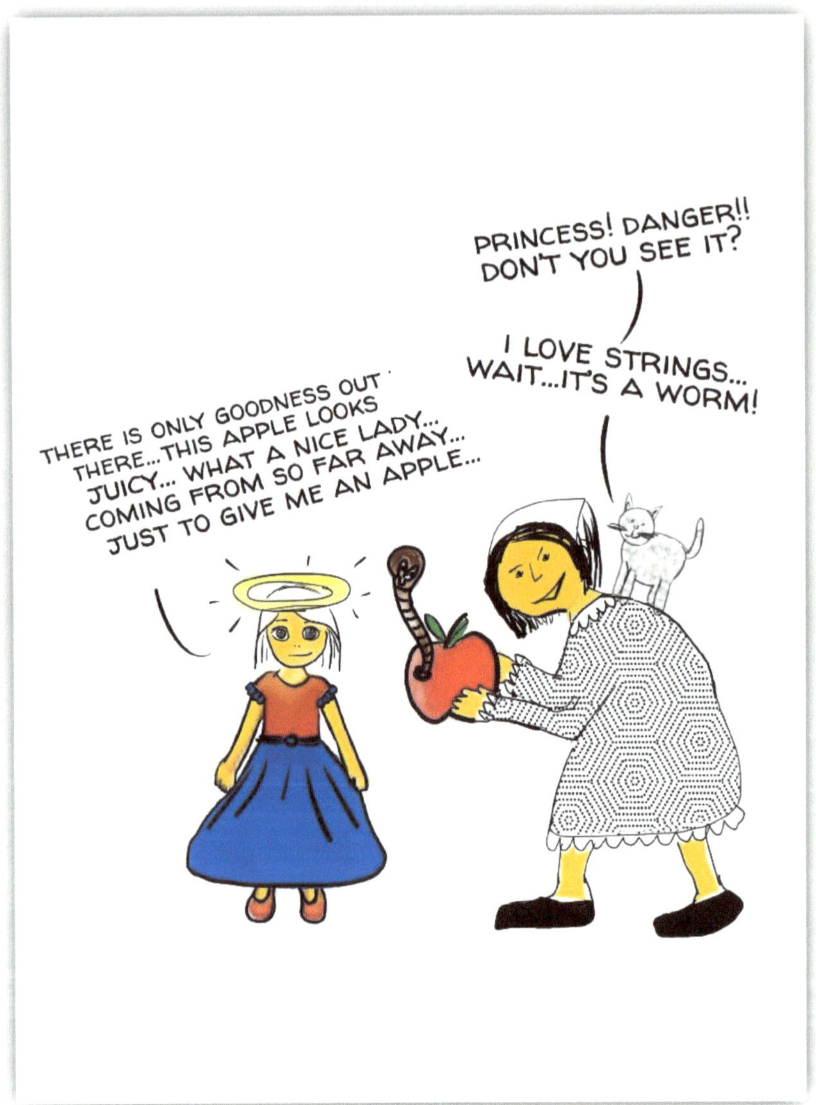

Homeopathic Fairy Tales:
Snow White

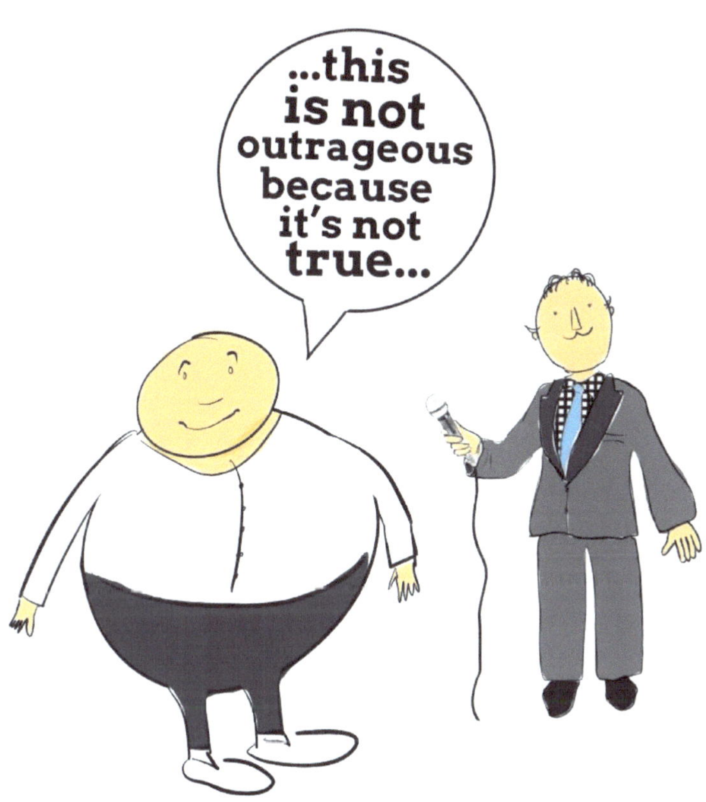
...this is not outrageous because it's not true...

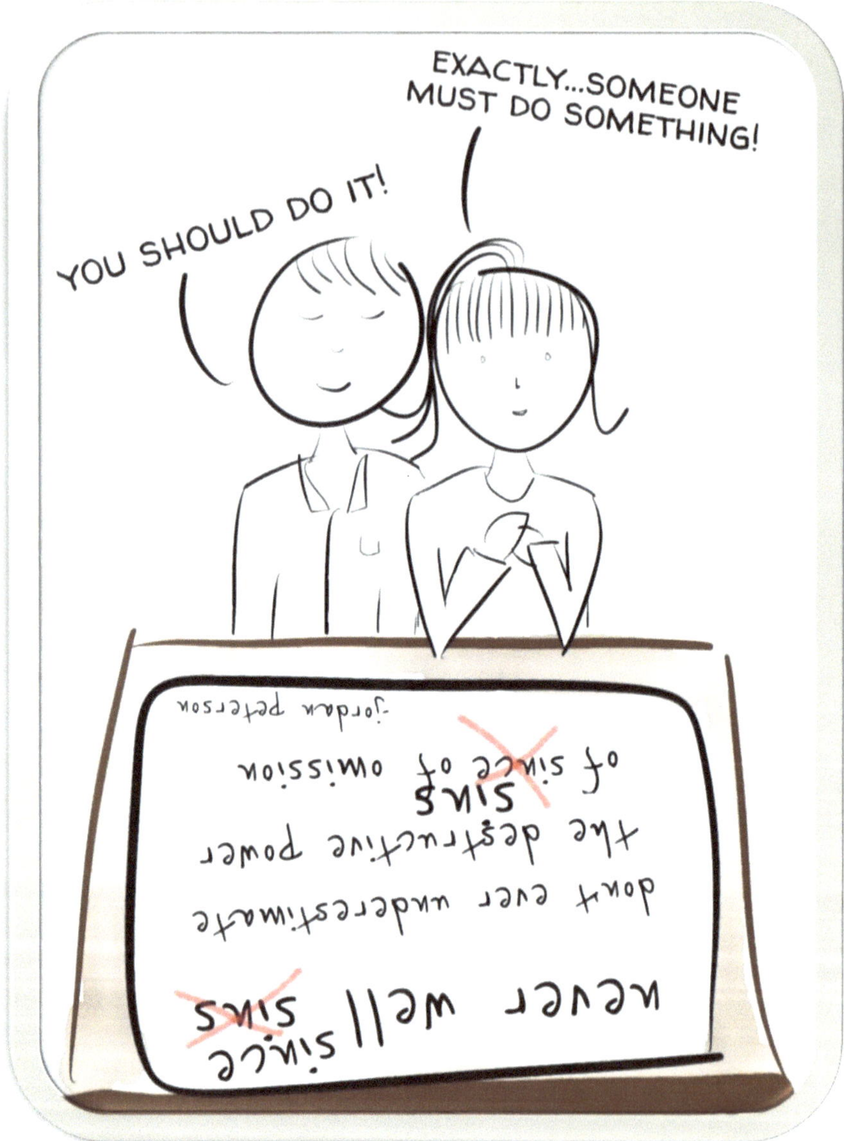
YOU SHOULD DO IT!
EXACTLY...SOMEONE MUST DO SOMETHING!
never well since
don't ever underestimate
the destructive power
of sins of omission
-jordan peterson

NWS

By Lena Kratz

NWS stands for *never well since* and is an important concept in homeopathy, but honestly, introducing it to all areas of medicine would make a lot of sense! NWS is an attempt to establish a timeline of events leading up to an illness. Anyone trying to set up such a timeline would be frequently surprised by its predictive powers and ability to pinpoint root causes of medical conditions. It is often possible to visualize a person's health by evaluating the presence or progression of certain risk factors—this way, serious events can often be foreseen and avoided for months, and, in some cases, perhaps for years. Sometimes it turns out that two seemingly unrelated events might be connected in a way which wasn't obvious before.

An experienced practitioner of alternative medicine can look at such a timeline and see the progression from eczema to asthma and then ADHD, for example. Even traumatic events, grief, or hardships, such as losing a job, can often be traced back in time as trigger points for physical ailments, making it possible to deal with the exact cause of the illness. Recognizing this type of NWS and addressing it often leads to great healing success.

Other NWSs could include long term effects of past serious injuries or chronic infections such as Lyme disease or mononucleosis.

The concept of NWS is based on the assumption that no one changes health levels suddenly for no reason—there must always be a trigger of some sort—emotional or physical. Getting ill out of nowhere is not something that is meant to happen.

But these days we cannot avoid hearing an awful lot of stories that go like this: the kids were happy, doing well through elementary school when suddenly, without warning—*crash!* —in 5th grade, their world fell apart!

Greta Thunberg, the teenage Swedish climate activist, is the latest prominent example of a classical NWS. Without going into her politics here, I think her personal story—just recently published as a book—is remarkable.[79] The family puts it this way: Greta's mother had been an opera singer, traveling the world with her family until Greta was in approximately 5th grade and *suddenly* developed a severe eating disorder. The parents spent months trying to pull her out of this hole, until coming up with the idea of engaging their daughter in an interesting project. While watching a movie about ecological disasters in school, Greta discovered her passion for environmental causes, specifically climate and environmental activism. Although she was barely able to avoid hospitalization and was later also diagnosed with Asperger's syndrome, depression, ADHD, and OCD—in addition to the eating disorder—the family managed to overcome the immediate crisis. Did they accomplish this just by distracting her from her health problems? Perhaps, but who knows—that is not the point here; it is entirely possible that Greta would have engaged in climate activism regardless of this emergency. The point is the unexpected suffering revealed by the story. Distress experienced not only by the child, but by the whole family was permeating their entire lives! And, as if this was not enough, the same thing happened a few years later to Greta's younger sister. Reaching the approximate age where Greta had fallen ill, she also began suffering from ADHD, Asperger's syndrome, and OCD. This kind of timeline is not for the faint hearted!

The procession of events raises eyebrows, the sudden onset of illness is puzzling. Predictably, comment sections about the Thunberg family's political activities are full of know-it-all opinions going both ways: "good for them, their courage is an inspiration!" or "I feel sorry for these people…" or "how dare they take a family crisis and turn it into a climate crisis! They are just trying to obscure their own problems…".

We don't know. It is best to be compassionate. But the comments are missing this important detail: it is highly unusual for healthy individuals to fall off a cliff in this way, without a trigger. There is almost certainly a NWS, especially because the same thing happened

[79] Ernman, M. and Thunberg, G. *Szenen aus dem Herzen*, Fischer, **2019**

to two children of the same family.

Some would argue that this is a perfect example for genetics to explain such outcomes—after all, two children who are blood related are affected almost equally. But the parents look alright and capable enough to me, raising the question of where it all came from. This doesn't appear to be a family with a complex mental health history—endless alcoholism or drug abuse, failure to achieve and child neglect—where such crises could be expected.

Nowadays school systems are constantly dealing with cases such as these.[80] A few years ago, the public middle school in our town sent out a letter, asking anyone with a strep throat to have it treated immediately in order to avoid spreading it, all because of certain cases of "very serious overreactions to strep bacteria". For the affected "overreacting" students, exposure to strep bacteria could be dangerous, causing them to develop sudden cases of anxiety and aggression, coupled with compulsive behavior.

As explained earlier, this sounds a lot like PANDAS to me. Similarly, another parent told us about the curious and scary case of a neighborhood girl who suddenly started suffering from OCD. The behavior change happened over night, "forcing" the child to constantly arrange and re-arrange her shoes and backpack. She wasn't "allowed" to touch a number of "forbidden" items and suffered from school anxiety.

Kids everywhere are developing eating disorders, low energy states, concentration problems, school anxiety, depression, tics, obsessions—you name it—*just over night!*

But it's not out of nowhere. It's not normal development either. It is a clear sign of sudden immune system damage, most likely a consequence of suppression and/or (un)necessary medical interventions. In the environment of an already chronically weak immune system, these interventions can create havoc. *Was this what had happened to us as a family, back when all our health problems had originally surfaced?* At least, it appears to be worth it to examine the impact of

[80] Maloney, B.A. *Saving Sammy, a mothers fight to cure her son's OCD* Three Rivers Press, New York **2009**

NWSs on our health histories—which brings us to the next section and some of the underlying reasons at the level of cellular dysfunction.

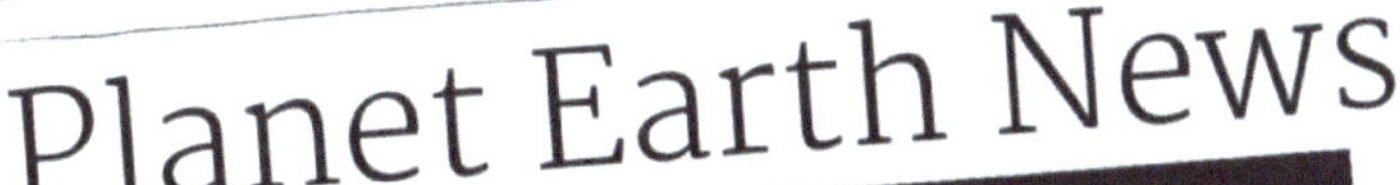

Planet Earth News

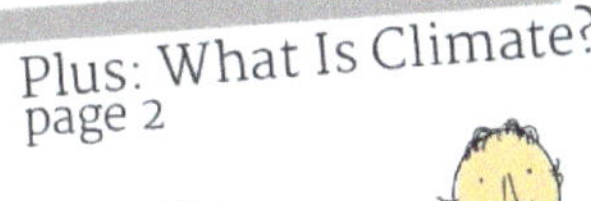

Plus: What Is Climate?
page 2

Greta Thunberg on planes, trains and sailboats page 5

Her Hopes For The Future: a chance for discussion at Mother Nature's party

****

Is it a NWS? Ms. Thunberg's struggles with Asperger's and eating disorders

Left it all behind? page 9

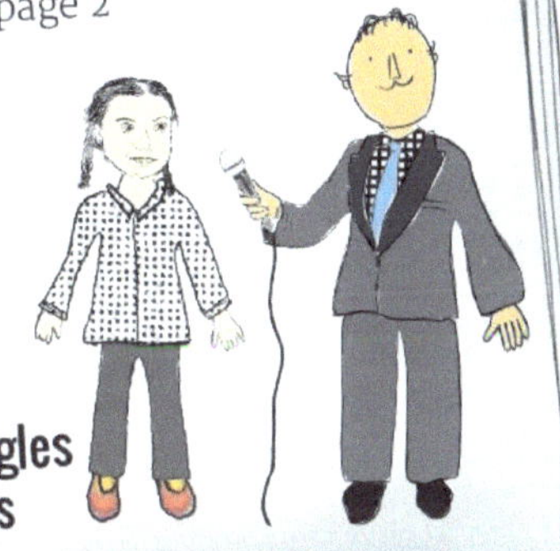

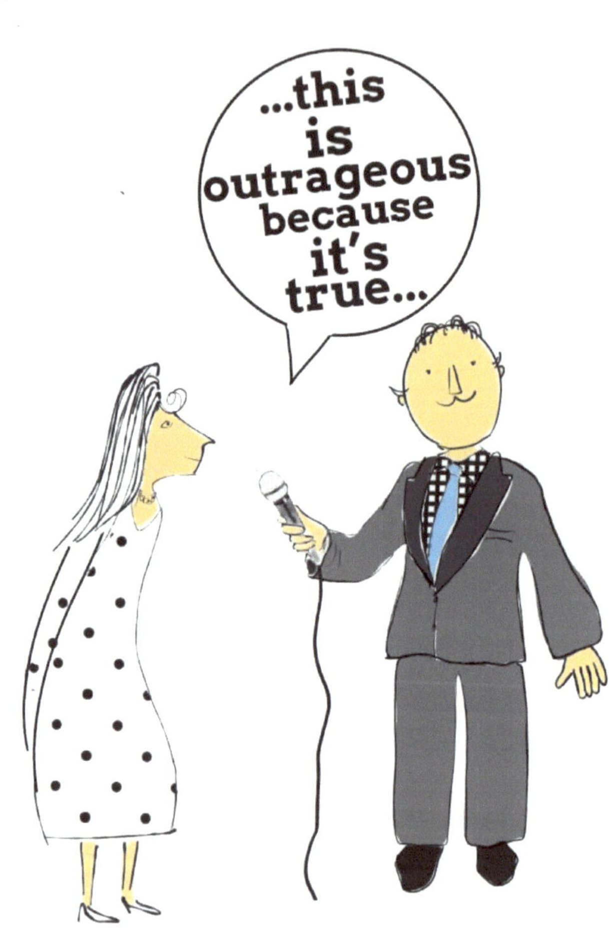
...this is outrageous because it's true...

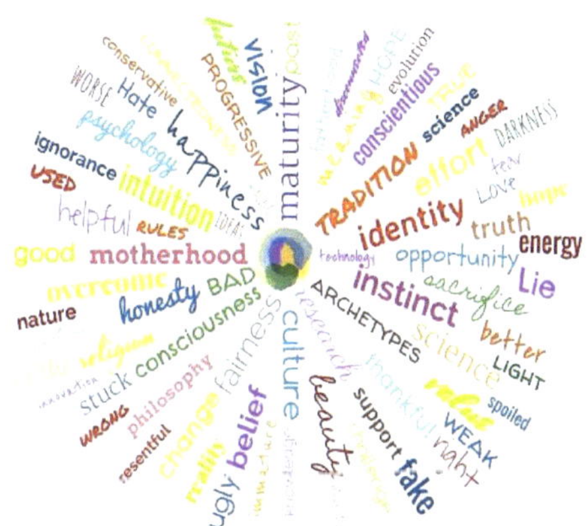
conservative
WORSE
Hate
psychology
ignorance
USED
intuition
helpful
RULES
good
motherhood
nature
honesty
BAD
consciousness
stuck
philosophy
WRONG
resentful
change
fairness
ugly
belief
culture
research
beauty
support
fake
night
WEAK
spoiled
LIGHT
better
science
ARCHETYPES
instinct
sacrifice
Lie
energy
opportunity
truth
identity
Love
TRADITION
effort
science
ANGER
DARKNESS
conscientious
evolution
HOPE
maturity
VISION
PROGRESSIVE
happiness
technology

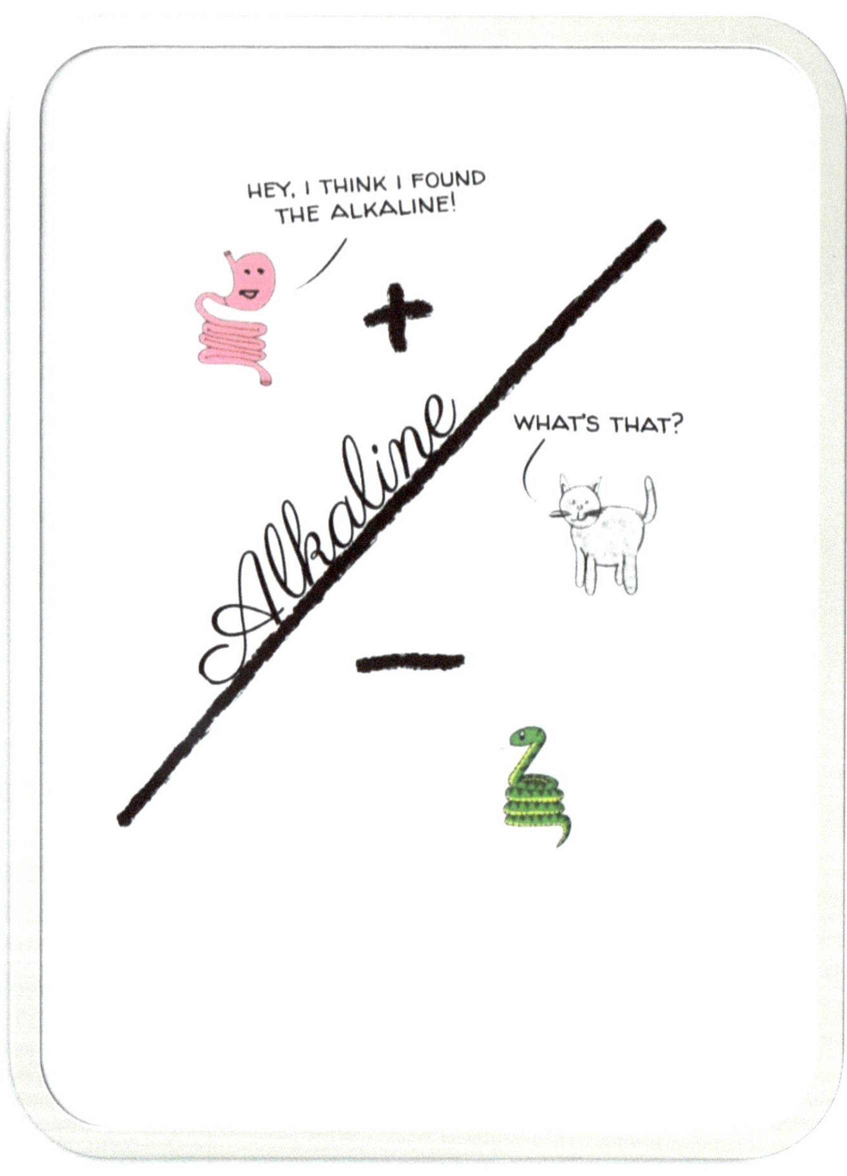
HEY, I THINK I FOUND THE ALKALINE!
+
Alkaline
WHAT'S THAT?
−

What in the World is Alkaline Water?

By Misna Burelli

As a chemist, I have been puzzled many times by health advertisements for "better" water, containing added baking soda. The baking soda is meant to push the pH of the water into the above seven region, making it alkaline. But then you swallow the water, letting it drop down into your stomach, which is filled with hydrochloric acid (HCl) with a pH of about two. That is really acidic, and the little speck of baking soda is no match. Besides, we want the stomach to be acidic—it helps to digest proteins and vitamin B12 containing foods.

Other food items such as fruits, nuts, legumes, and vegetables are also often marketed this way—by promising to alkalize the body. So, what's the point? Is there any truth to these beliefs? It took me a while to sort out what's going on, prompting me to take a journey to the unexpected places of cell biology and water.

According to the book *Healing is Voltage*, by Jerry Tennant,[81] all cells in our bodies are supposed to run at a voltage between minus 20 mV to minus 50 mV, depending on the task at hand. The creation of new cells needs the higher potential of minus 50 mV, while everyday metabolism needs only about minus 20 mV to minus 25 mV. Repairs are also done at the higher potential of minus 50 mV, and can only be successfully completed if the potential stays at that level long enough to replace the damaged parts.

Now imagine your body's voltage dropping back into the minus 20 mV range before all repairs are completed—it's like unfinished homework piling up somewhere. Any patch-up that gets delayed will become chronic, simply because we did not solve the problem. Chronic problems tend to pass through a cycle of flaring up, fading away, and then returning with renewed intensity—but *never resolving* completely. The only exception to this rule occurs for true healing—a period of prolonged inflammation that is followed by no inflammation—because the problem has been solved.

[81] Tennantinstitute.com, Tenant, J. *Healing is Voltage*, **2013**

We don't see this happening very often, but when it does occur, the inflammation giving rise to healing can be painfully noticeable. In what is called "return of old symptoms", these old wounds act up, responding to previously unsuccessful attempts at fixing the problem. The uncomfortable symptoms are a sign that the body is mounting an actual effort to repair a bunch of broken parts. Therefore, the return of old symptoms is nothing more than the body getting a boost from somewhere, reaching the right cell voltage required for repairs, and healing what needs to be healed!

Unfortunately, most of the time we don't experience a return of old symptoms because our bodies gave up; unable to generate the necessary voltage, we now accept living with whatever chronic ailment replaced the acute condition we failed to repair.

So, how about just increasing the "repair voltage"? How can we even tell that we don't have enough healing "potential" in our body? Simple: we can measure the pH inside and outside of our cells to calculate the cross-membrane potential. The pH—which is the negative logarithm of the hydronium ion concentration in an aqueous solution—is really a measure of voltage where the abbreviation pH stands for "potential hydrogen". A pH of 7 is neutral. A pH above 7 is alkaline, and a pH below 7 is acidic.

So, what is the optimum potential we are looking for? On a scale of pH 0-14, an acidic pH of 0 equals plus 400 mV, a neutral pH of 7 equals 0 mV, and an alkaline pH of 14 equals minus 400 mV. A typical cell repair pH of 7.88 would equal minus 50 mV, and a normal everyday cell pH of 7.44 would equal minus 25 mV. It comes down to this: any aqueous solution with a negative millivolt readout is an electron donor, while one resulting in a positive millivolt measurement is an electron stealer. Our cells are designed to run under electron donor conditions.

There are a lot of indications from Dr. Tennant's private research and personal experiences to assume that a cell pH of less than the normal 7.44 means big trouble: as the pH drops, draining us of energy, we first get tired, before getting sick and unable to repair any damage or heal any chronic condition. At pH 7 we switch polarity—*there is that word again!* At a pH of less than 7—slightly acidic—we are drifting toward cancer.

So, no wonder everyone is always looking to "alkalize" their system, although it has nothing to do with baking soda in drinking water. What we really need is a reliable method to recharge our cells when they are depleted.

This theory matches well with other observations, both from homeopathy and mainstream research, suggesting that cancer is a low oxygen state.[82] In an acidic state, as the pH of the body drops, oxygen cannot be dissolved properly within our body. The resulting low oxygen state affects the conversion of glucose to carbon dioxide and water—it is no longer possible to burn glucose with insufficient oxygen—forcing the implementation of an altered energy metabolism. Is this the reason why some cancer cells have their energy producing mitochondria altered or switched off? And this is also where we find a connection to our sugar metabolism.[83] Switching off a cell's mitochondria compels it to produce energy through anaerobic—no oxygen—respiration, generating lactic acid, and ramping up sugar consumption, as energy production becomes much less efficient.

A lowered cell pH, with its concomitant low oxygen state, is also linked to the obesity epidemic plaguing the world. Detoxification, usually taking place through oxidation, is exceedingly difficult to achieve in a low oxygen environment. As a result, the body is forced to do the next best thing: *storing the toxins*, usually in a chunk of fat produced just for that purpose. Have you seen obese people who are constantly hungry, claiming their faulty body signals are directing them to eat inappropriately? These are no faulty signals leading them astray! Running out of detoxification capacity, the body is just ordering additional toxin storage in the form of fat—which makes them hungry! Dieting invariably leads to the opening of those toxin storage units, therefore often producing an intolerable state of detoxification symptoms. As the low oxygen body environment is overwhelmed, these symptoms are

---

[82] Muz, B. et al. The role of hypoxia in cancer progression, angiogenesis, metastasis, and resistance to therapy *Hypoxia*, **2015**, *3*:83-92

[83] Zeviar, D.D. et al. The Role of Mitochondria in Cancer and Other Chronic Diseases *JOM* **2014**, *29(4)*:157-166

often so difficult to bear that the diet fails.

It is a similar story for infections. Bacteria, fungi or parasites cannot be effectively countered without oxygen—this is how the body's defense system works! Dropping oxygen levels might set the stage for chronic infections to flare up, or for dormant parasites to take over. Bugs that were mostly under control in a high oxygen environment will wake up the moment the oxygen levels drop, setting the stage for serious disease to commence. This can occur rather quickly. Is that what happens to children waking up with PANDAS one day, or in many of the previously discussed cases of NWS?

Relaxing in oxygen chambers has become a popular procedure in alternative medicine, alleviating certain conditions just by improving detoxification and energy metabolism.[84] But, of course, it does not solve the fundamental problem of low cell oxygen, due to a low pH and a faulty cell membrane potential.

Also consider this, the next time you are loading up on "antioxidants". It is true that humans are an anomaly when it comes to the production of vitamin C, one of the primary antioxidants in our bodies. Most mammals, except for guinea pigs and humans, can produce their own vitamin C when sick. Goats, for example, can synthesize up to 100g of it per day. But what does it do with it? That is less clear. Publications and reports of miracle cures by vitamin C-IV-treatment have been all over alternative health news for a long time. Famous Nobel Prize winner Linus Pauling endorsed the concept in the 90's, consuming up to 13 g of vitamin C per day—making it tempting to advocate for such treatments without question. Since curing anything is complicated business, I will not get into the details of approving or discrediting anyone here—after all, Linus Pauling lived to the ripe old age of 94—but rather just throw in this question: if most detoxification is done by oxidizing, is it always an advantage to constantly and permanently fill yourself up with antioxidants? After all, the goat seems to produce large amounts of vitamin C only during acute illness, making it reasonable to

---

[84] Conroy, H. et al. *The Thinking Moms' Revolution: Autism beyond the Spectrum: Inspiring True Stories from Parents Fighting to Rescue Their Children*, Skyhorse, **2013**

assume that high, long-term intake of antioxidants might not always be desirable.

James Watson, another Nobel Prize winner and one of the discoverers of the double helix structure of DNA, is a critic of the overconsumption of antioxidants. In an article called "cancer manifesto",[85] he points out the roles of oxidants and antioxidants in the human body, and the fact that a faulty oxygen metabolism and dysfunctional mitochondria are related to cancer. As mentioned earlier, some antiparasitic drugs, such as mebendazole, have been repurposed as cancer treatments, highlighting the possible connections between chronic parasite infections, low cellular oxygen levels, and cancer.

Even though it seems like antioxidants could help with recharging our cells, by preventing unnecessary electron loss, there is obviously a place for oxidation in energy metabolism, detoxification, and the immune system as a whole. The process of oxidation is just isolated well from areas it could damage. So, it seems that we are back to pondering the same question again: maybe *both poles are necessary*? After all, a higher negative cell voltage, which is the same as a higher cell pH, leads to a higher cellular oxygen level, therefore automatically providing both sides of the spectrum.

At this moment, research provides no quick answers to such questions, but one thing is clear: we need a reliable way to recharge our cells, a method of introducing negative ions into the body, without interfering with our oxygen metabolism.

So, what are the options? Healthy, fresh vegetables and unprocessed meals provide electrons in the form of natural antioxidants, while walking barefoot on grass conducts the earth's electricity straight into the body—yes, our planet is a large electron donor! To make up for this century's unhealthy indoor lifestyles, it is now possible to buy "grounding" products: "grounding shoes", "grounding sheets" for beds and "grounding mats" for computer desks. These products just plug into the grounding outlets of electrical sockets or have a direct connection to the soil outside. A similar invention aims to detoxify the body through

---

[85] Watson, J. Oxidants, antioxidants and the current incurability of metastatic cancers *Open Biology*, **2013**, *Vol 3(1)*

ionic foot baths.

The goal of all these products is to improve a poor cell membrane potential by introducing negative ions directly into cells. But it is more complicated than just adding electrons: our cell membranes must be able to *hold* the charge, by acting as "capacitors". A typical cell membrane is constructed of layers of conducting and insulating materials—*creating a capacitor*—and the quality of the building materials is crucial!

Watching what we eat becomes ever more important in this time of unnatural and fake dietary choices, as trans fats and rancid oils are inadequate to serve as membrane building blocks. We need unmodified, natural, saturated, and unsaturated fats, for the insulating parts of our cell membranes to build well working cell membrane capacitors.

To make matters more complicated, we can look at the cross membrane potential in another way—from the point of view of the molecular biologists who came up with the theory of the sodium-potassium pump.[86] It has been generally accepted knowledge that this pump is mainly responsible for the aforementioned charge distribution across the cell wall. It has been a paradigm.

But in 2001, a scientist named Gilbert Ling put a dent into this paradigm by calculating the pump's energy requirements.[87] After a little bit of math, he came to the conclusion that such a pump was an unrealistic proposal; about fifteen to thirty times more energy was needed to run the pump than is reasonably available. That's a lot—if correct, there is no way for a cell to come up with this kind of energy.

In addition, his other experiments literally poked holes into the ion pump theory by showing that cells could be punctured with micropipettes without any effect on the charge gradient of the cell membrane. They also never leaked—holes in the walls didn't seem to matter much.

The topic was picked up by Gerald Pollack, who proposed that water has four phases: solid, liquid, gas and gel. This newly discovered gel-like fourth phase of water was speculated to automatically carry a

---

[86] Swedish scientist Jens Christian Skou in 1950

[87] Ling, G. *Life at the Cell and Below-Cell Level*, Pacific Press **2001**

negative charge, while its semi-solid consistency provided a mesh-like medium, capable of catching potassium ions, while excluding sodium ions. The observed cell gradient would simply be a result of exclusion of one type of ion versus another—no pumps needed. More scientific background can be found in Pollack's book, *The Fourth Phase of Water: Beyond Solid, Liquid, Vapor*, which is available in many public libraries.[88]

The idea of a fourth phase of water provides us with an additional option to charge our cells—by drinking water mostly in this fourth phase, freshly energized by Mother Nature. This water would have been spinning and tumbling over rocks, absorbing the Earth's energy. Of course, no one has time to hike to their favorite waterfall in the morning, so Pollack has been busy designing water filters that mimic the action of waterfalls—maybe we should all have our own personal waterfall at home!

[88] Pollack, G.H. *The Fourth Phase of Water: Beyond Solid, Liquid, Vapor* Seattle Ebner and Sons Publishing, **2013**

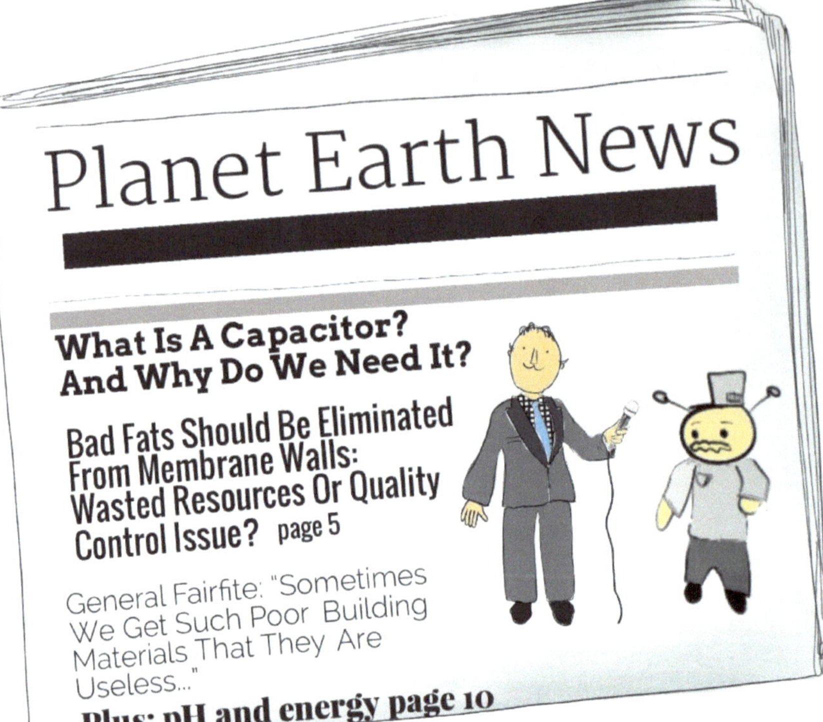
Planet Earth News

What Is A Capacitor?
And Why Do We Need It?

Bad Fats Should Be Eliminated From Membrane Walls: Wasted Resources Or Quality Control Issue? page 5

General Fairfite: "Sometimes We Get Such Poor Building Materials That They Are Useless..."

Plus: pH and energy page 10

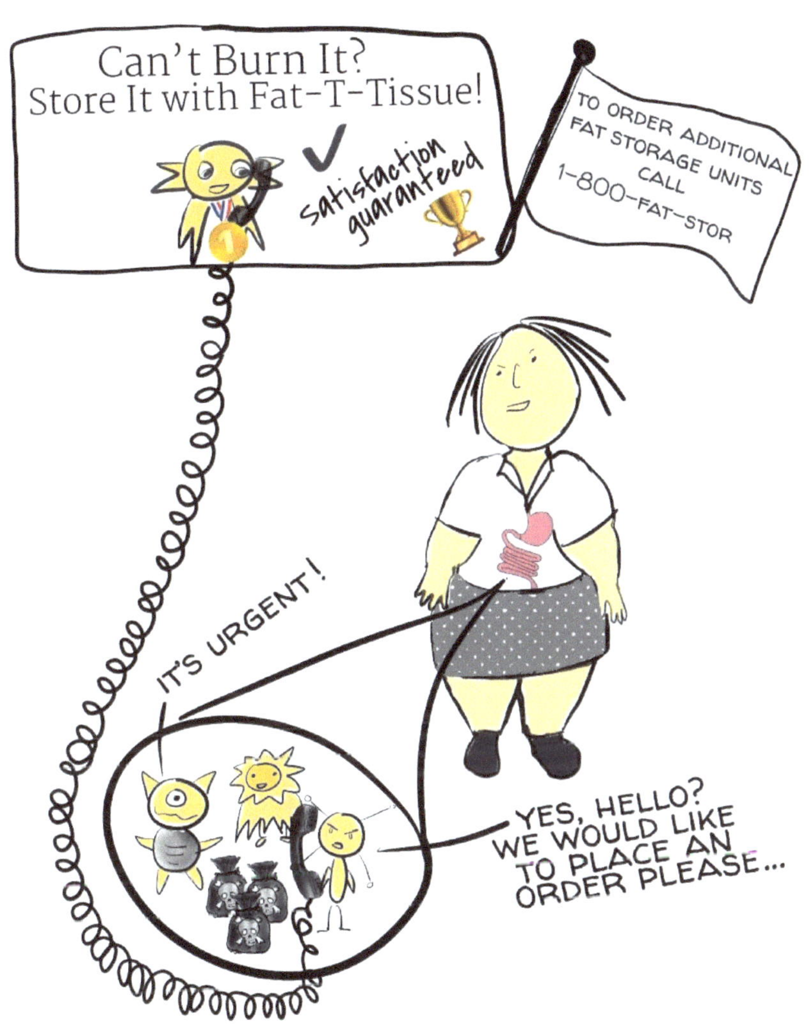
Can't Burn It?
Store It with Fat-T-Tissue!
satisfaction guaranteed
TO ORDER ADDITIONAL FAT STORAGE UNITS CALL
1-800-FAT-STOR
IT'S URGENT!
YES, HELLO?
WE WOULD LIKE TO PLACE AN ORDER PLEASE...

SCIENCE CAN NEVER BE SETTLED...
WHEN SCIENCE IS SETTLED...
IT BECOMES A RELIGION...

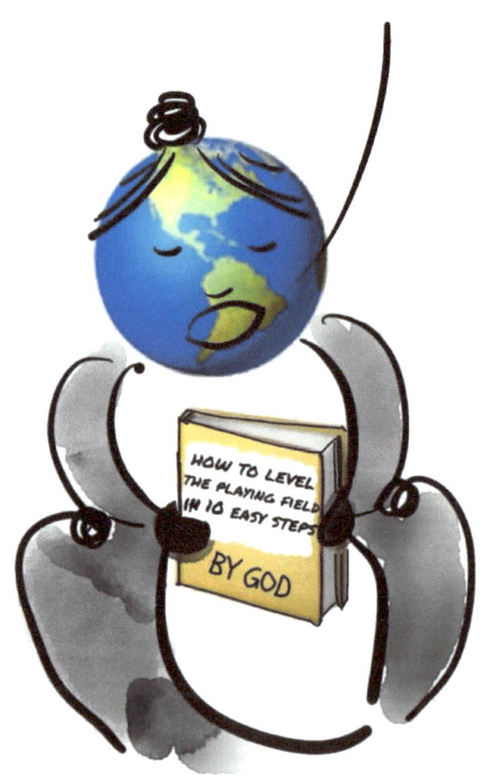

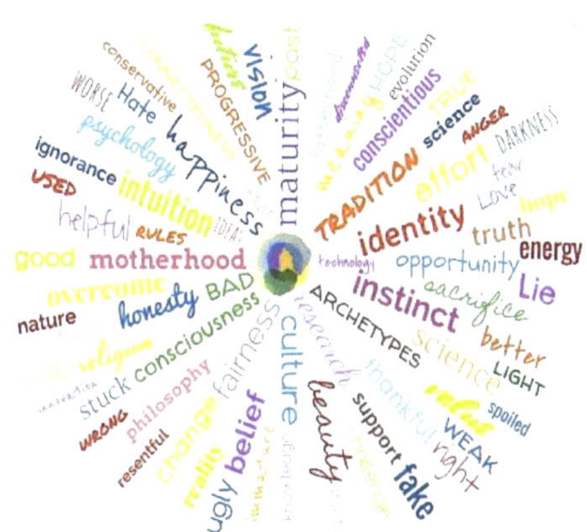
conservative
WORSE
Hate
psychology
happiness
PROGRESSIVE
VISION
maturity
past
evolution
HOPE
conscientious
TRUE
science
ANGER
DARKNESS
ignorance
USED
intuition
TRADITION
effort
fear
Love
hope
helpful
RULES
identity
truth
energy
good
motherhood
technology
opportunity
overcome
honesty
BAD
instinct
sacrifice
Lie
nature
ARCHETYPES
better
religion
consciousness
science
LIGHT
stuck
philosophy
fairness
culture
research
thankful
spoiled
WRONG
resentful
change
belief
beauty
support
WEAK
right
reality
ugly
fake

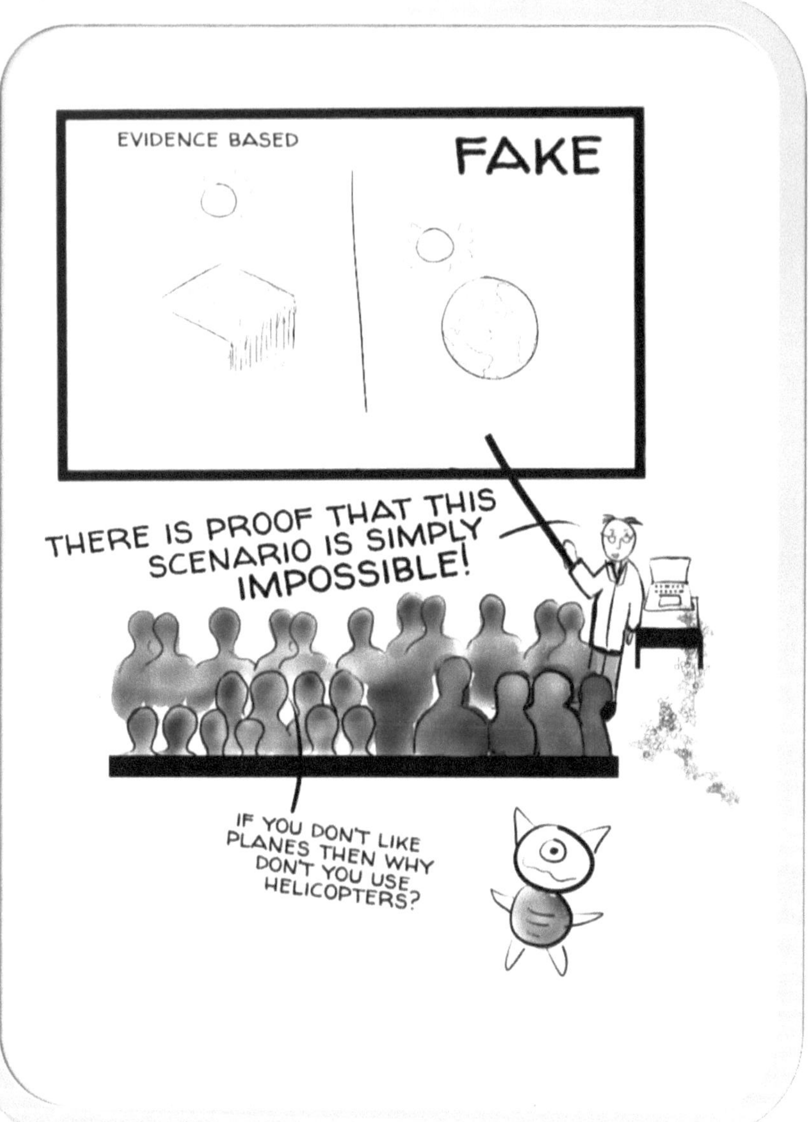
EVIDENCE BASED
FAKE
THERE IS PROOF THAT THIS SCENARIO IS SIMPLY IMPOSSIBLE!
IF YOU DON'T LIKE PLANES THEN WHY DON'T YOU USE HELICOPTERS?

In Desperate Need of Real Research

By Lena Kratz

I love research—but where has it gone?

Our chemistry department came together for a fancy retirement gathering. People flew in from everywhere, with many guests from Europe and Asia. It was the usual: speeches by former graduate students, jokes about working every weekend, and the highlights and pitfalls of their own careers, now that they were professors or directors somewhere.

My former lab mates, our professor, her husband, and I were sat around a dinner table, chatting. Next to me, a former graduate student, who was now working at a large pharmaceutical company, talked about life as a pharma industry researcher. It took me a while—but then I decided to disclose my interest in alternative medicine. One former lab mate, a mother of three, seemed curious but unsure of what to say—others had started looking irritated. I wasn't supposed to say things like this! My professor's husband, who was not a chemist, chimed in that he had heard of great success stories in the alternative medicine field—awkward silence.

We changed topics and started talking about our families. I asked a former classmate about his son's career plans. His son was almost graduating from high school, but all he revealed was "he still has a lot to learn". I dug a little deeper and found out that "the only thing that he's interested in is football… but he's not good enough at that. At this moment he doesn't have many other ambitions, but we hope that he will find himself. He's probably just a little immature". It sounded like he had tried to figure out what was wrong with his son but couldn't. A Ph.D. chemist, working successfully in the pharma industry, making good amounts of money, somehow had a kid who wasn't interested in anything—this kind of scenario has become absolutely common. Everywhere you go, you will hear the key words "finding himself" and "immature".

Even though, at this point, I could have talked a lot about

alternative healthcare, archetypes and our own personal journey, I sensed that I had no audience, so I stayed quiet.

The evening ended with small talk only, and I felt seriously out of place in that crowd, even though I had completely belonged to it only a few years ago. But why was I so afraid of speaking up, of having a true discussion? It was because I had no arguments. Homeopathy was considered to be a placebo, a known "side effect" of believing in a helpful medication. There was no solid proof anywhere in the literature that homeopathy worked in any other way or what its alternative mechanism of action could be, beyond the placebo effect. In this circle here, even diet research was suspect. *Yeah, not a chance.*

Another friend from my former workplace was more open and—upon my recommendation—tried some alternative health care for her daughter, who was suffering from a range of severe food allergies, including a dangerous peanut allergy. It was a halfhearted attempt that led nowhere, but at least she wasn't completely opposed, and I'm still good friends with her. She also has a very successful career in the pharma field.

I heard more stories through gossip: the son of one of Misna's friends came home from college during freshman year, only to sit in the basement of his parents' house, playing video games. What had happened to that child?

The exact opposite, yet the same, took place at homeopathy graduation: several people gave speeches, talking about fancy archetypes, going back to the old fire, water, air, and earth element theory and in the end, everyone got a graduation diploma. We all shared a little bit of our vision— where we would be going with this newfound knowledge. Most of us would just be trying to help people individually—nothing wrong with that. And for the most part, there were enough customers. What else was there to do? Our field was tiny and not well accepted. I was more or less the only one with a science background in that crowd, making it impossible to discuss matters such as homeopathic mechanisms of action. In a strange sort of way, I was out of place again. When it was my turn to speak, I announced that for me the most important thing was to research homeopathy—to find out how it worked! It wasn't an attention-grabber. But then people started saying things like "good for you, we need someone like that…good luck!" and, "I have an email of someone else who is interested in this". I asked, "would you like to join me?" No one would.

Both of these scenarios illustrate the total disconnect between "regular mainstream science" and "alternative science". Alternative practitioners are simply tired as a result of constantly having to defend themselves, justifying their very existence. If most mainstream scientists believe that even healing through diet is on the level of conspiracy theories—unless, of course, using official low-fat dietary guidelines—common ground is difficult to find, while stepping outside the box is impossible.

No matter where you go, it's only mainstream messages: I have seen friends boil eggs, sincerely explaining to their children the nutritional benefits of the white part, whereas condemning the yolk to the trash can in an attempt to reduce the family's cholesterol. Never mind the vastly superior vitamin and fat content of the egg yolk—vitamins and fats which could be used to build excellent cell membrane capacitors! Such extreme positions are irrational and should be avoided, but often such matters cannot even be discussed without creating controversy. Imagine what other topics can't be touched at all! Unfortunately, this attitude of dodging certain contentious issues grows out of fear of not being taken seriously. It might be career damaging to engage in "unscientific" discussions—no one wants to be discredited this way, so no one dares to go there.

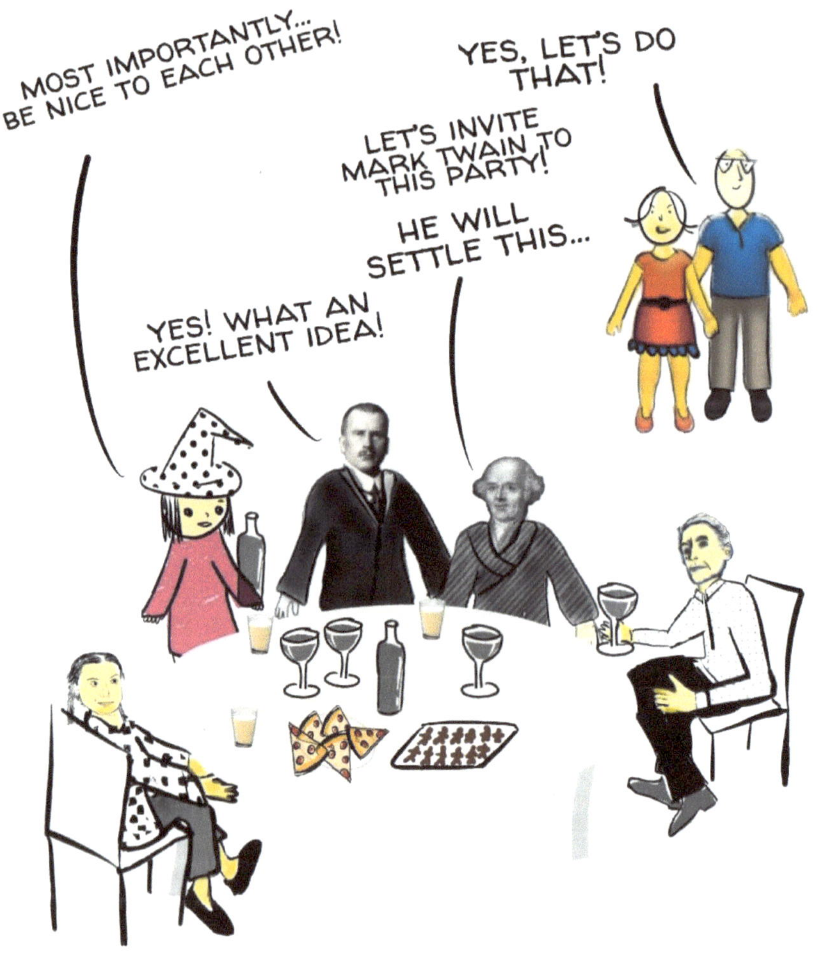
MOST IMPORTANTLY...
BE NICE TO EACH OTHER!
YES! WHAT AN
EXCELLENT IDEA!
HE WILL
SETTLE THIS...
LET'S INVITE
MARK TWAIN TO
THIS PARTY!
YES, LET'S DO
THAT!

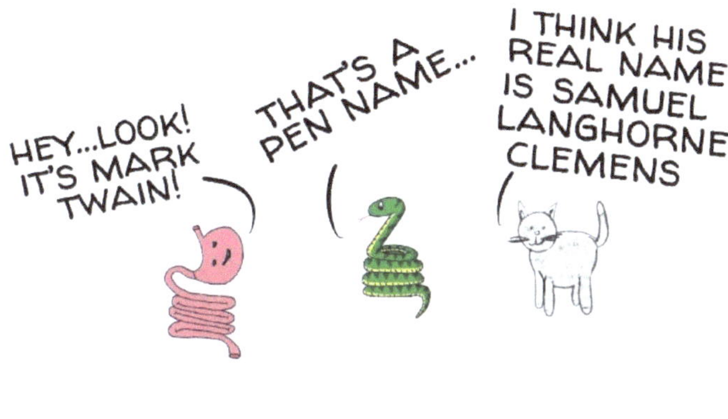
HEY...LOOK! IT'S MARK TWAIN!
THAT'S A PEN NAME...
I THINK HIS REAL NAME IS SAMUEL LANGHORNE CLEMENS

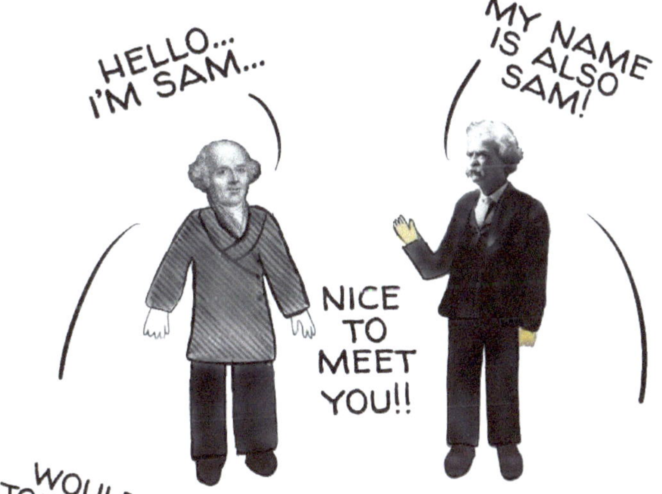
HELLO... I'M SAM...
MY NAME IS ALSO SAM!
NICE TO MEET YOU!!
WOULD YOU LIKE TO JOIN US AT THE PARTY?
SURE, WHY NOT?

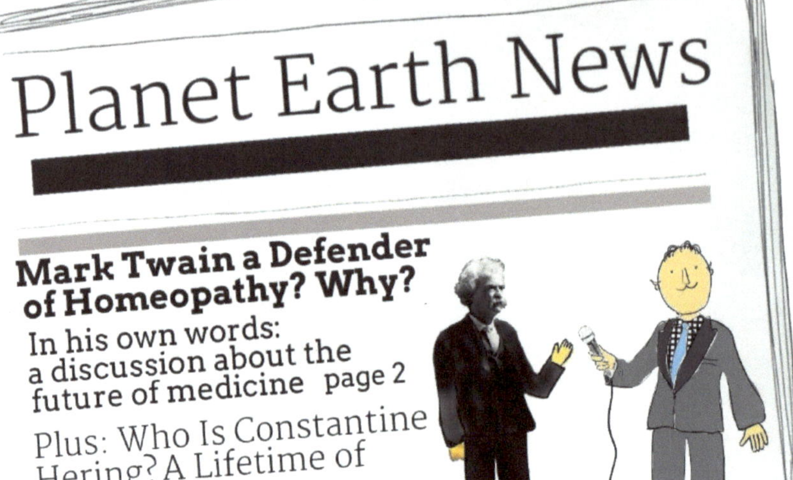
Planet Earth News
Mark Twain a Defender of Homeopathy? Why?
In his own words: a discussion about the future of medicine page 2
Plus: Who Is Constantine Hering? A Lifetime of Service page 5
Hahnemann University Hospital in Philadelphia to close September 2019

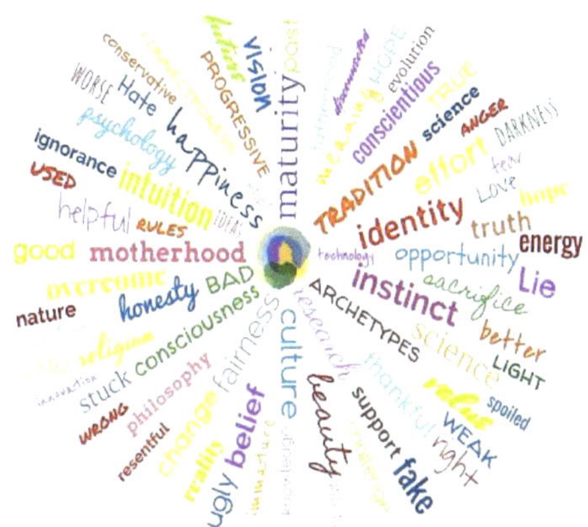
maturity
identity
truth
energy
opportunity
Lie
instinct
sacrifice
better
LIGHT
ARCHETYPES
science
spoiled
WEAK
support
fake
beauty
culture
research
fairness
belief
ugly
change
philosophy
resentful
WRONG
stuck
consciousness
honesty
BAD
nature
good
motherhood
helpful
RULES
intuition
USED
ignorance
psychology
Hate
WORSE
conservative
happiness
PROGRESSIVE
VISION
TRADITION
effort
LOVE
DARKNESS
ANGER
science
conscientious
evolution
technology

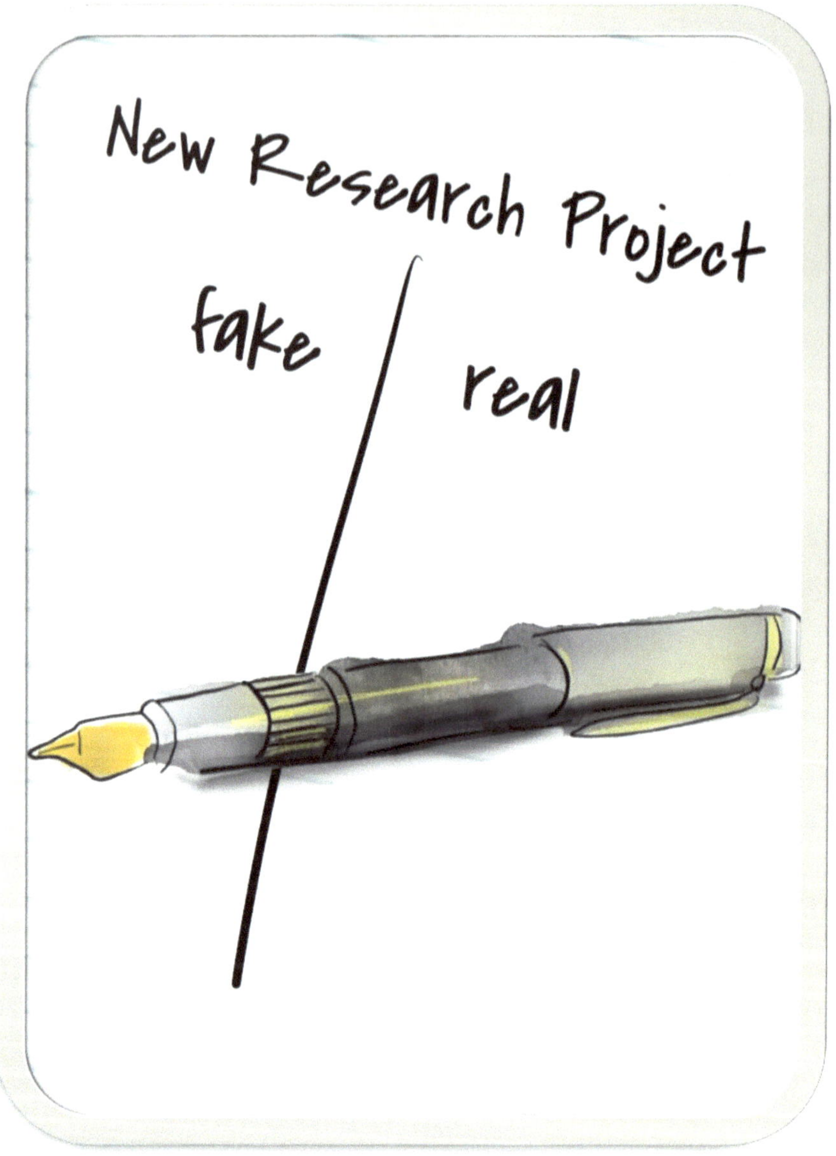
New Research Project
fake
real

But I Did It Anyway

By Misna Burelli

There was only one option: we needed to find out how homeopathy works—its mechanism of action, current applications, and future research opportunities. In short: we needed a solid theory that was easily defendable. So, we set out doing exactly that, against all common sense and while working at a full-time job. Lena was worried that it would be too much, and even now, I admit she was not completely wrong about that.

My first step involved scanning all the literature, looking for foreign—mostly Indian—contributions, and going from there. I discovered that the Banerji family's large Kolkata homeopathic medical clinic had lots of collaborations with The University of Texas MD Anderson Cancer Center. Their research protocol was even included in a United States (US) National Cancer Institute (NCI) Best Case Series (BCS) Program,[89] and was found worthy of follow up, due to good results.

Other research came from Switzerland,[90] including a clinical trial using homeopathy to improve ADHD symptoms in children.[91] Unfortunately, the extremely promising data sort of "fizzled out" when the crossover started.[92] A controlled trial environment is not a good match for homeopathy, especially when treating chronic conditions like ADHD. Homeopathy is based on archetypes, not one-size-fits-all medicine, making it difficult to compare outcomes using the same

[89] Banerji, P.; Campbell, D.R. and Banerji, P. Cancer patients treated with the Banerji protocols utilizing homeopathic medicine: a Best Case Series Program of the National Cancer Institute USA *Oncol. Rep.* **2008**, *20(1)*:69-74

[90] Frei, H. et al. Treatment for hyperactive children: homeopathy and methylphenidate compared in a family setting *Br. Homeopath. J.* **2001**, *90(4)*:183-8

[91] Frei, H. Homeopathic treatment of children with attention deficit hyperactivity disorder: a randomized, double blind, placebo controlled crossover trial *Eur. J. Pediatr.* **2005**, *164(12)*:758-67

[92] Frei, H. Randomised controlled trials of homeopathy in hyperactive children: treatment procedure leads to an unconventional study design. Experience with open-label homeopathic treatment preceding the Swiss ADHD placebo controlled, randomized, double-blind, crossover trial *Homeopathy* **2007**, *96(1)*:35-41

remedy or dose. On top of that, there are lots of variables: archetypes could be poorly selected, leading to failure in some cases and success in others, or unexpected changes after a remedy adjustment.

Other literature claimed that homeopathy improved arthritis symptoms; however, the effect was not due to the remedy, but rather the consultation.[93] *How did they know?*

Treating simple, acute conditions like injuries and diarrheal diseases—this also included surgeries and facelifts—showed the most promising results, with the most improved outcomes.[94] But none of it had anything to do with a mechanism of action.

Then there was one article discussing differences between certain types of homeopathic aqueous solutions and controls analyzed by expensive analytical instruments such as NMR. This was more interesting, as the authors claimed that they saw something there—a difference between the two solutions.[95]

I dived into more far-out territory and came across articles like "Metal nanoparticles induced hermetic activation: a novel mechanism of homeopathic medicines",[96] "Electromagnetic and magnetic vector potential bio-information and water",[97] and finally "Conscience and consciousness: a definition",[98] written by well-known homeopath George Vithoulkas. There was even an article about homeopathy and

[93] Brien, S. et al Homeopathy has clinical benefits in rheumatoid arthritis patients that are attributable to the consultation process but not the homeopathic remedy: a randomized controlled trial *Rheumatology* (Oxford), **2011**, *50(6):*1070-82

[94] Jacobs, J. Homeopathy for childhood diarrhea: combined results and metaanalysis from three randomized, controlled clinical trials *Pediatr. Infect. Dis. J.* **2003**, *22(3):*229-34

[95] Van Wasserhosen, M. et al. Nuclear Magnetic Resonance characterization of traditional homeopathically manufactured copper (Cuprum metallicum) and plant (Gelsemium sempervirens) medicines and controls *Homeopathy* **2017**, *106(4):*223-239

[96] Chikramane, P.S. et al. Metal nanoparticle induced hormetic activation: a novel mechanism of homeopathic medicines *Homeopathy* **2017**, *106(3):*135-144

[97] Smith, C.W. Electromagnetic and magnetic vector potential bio-information and water *Homeopathy*, **2015**, *104(4):*301-4

[98] Vithoulkas, G. et al. Conscience and consciousness: a definition *J. Med. Life* **2014**, *7(1):*104-8

string theory,[99] and many more[100] [101] [102] about quantum theories.[103]

These kinds of articles were similar to the ones published by the Queen's former homeopathic physician, Peter Fisher,[104] who had been tragically killed in a bicycle accident in London in 2018.[105]

And yes, it seems to me that he has done a good job treating the queen while she was under his care—at the age of ninety-three, she's still fulfilling her duties with competence, displaying an energy that many younger people simply have to admire.

Are you surprised that she would choose homeopathy? Just in case you thought that this was a chance occurrence, an example far outside the norm for rich and powerful people, consider Dana Ullman's book which is titled *The Homeopathic Revolution: Why Famous People and Cultural Heroes Choose Homeopathy*.[106] In it, he presents lists of names of people that we all recognize from sports, acting, or politics—rich and famous people who couldn't live without homeopathy. *Just sayin'…I wouldn't want you to miss out…*

Another interesting detail has been the number of hospitals that had been homeopathic, usually during the 1800s, prior to being converted to mainstream. There must have been a reason for a theory fresh out of Europe to catch on to the extent of converting the majority of regular hospitals into homeopathic research facilities, including homeopathic professorships, chairs, and faculty.

---

99 https://hpathy.com/scientific-research/string-theory-homoeopathy/

100 Rutten, L. et al. Plausibility and evidence: the case of homeopathy *Med. Health Care Philos.* **2013**, *16(3):*525-32

101 Milagros, L.R. The vital force "reincarnated": modeling entelechy as a quantized spinning gyroscopic metaphor for integrated medicine *Adv. Exp. Med. Biol.* **2015,** *821:*111-23

102 Thomas, Y. From high dilutions to digital biology: the physical nature of the biological signal *Homeopathy* **2015**, *104(4):*295-300

103 Manzalini, A. et al. Explaining Homeopathy with Quantum Electrodynamics *Homeopathy* **2019**, in print

104 Fisher, P. Is quantum entanglement in homeopathy a reality? *Homeopathy* **2016**, *105(3):*209-210

105 https://www.independent.co.uk/news/uk/home-news/dr-peter-fisher-dead-queen-homeopathic-doctor-london-cyclist-deaths-lorry-crushed-homeopathy-a8494456.html

106 Ullman, D. *The Homeopathic Revolution: Why Famous People and Cultural Heroes Choose Homeopathy*, **2007**

Many of these hospitals are still around today, even operating under the same homeopathic name—often Hahnemann—but without homeopathic treatments. There is a Hahnemann Campus at UMass Memorial Medical center, hinting at its homeopathic past. And Hahnemann University Hospital in Philadelphia has just been in the news regarding its bankruptcy and a plan to move about 570 resident physicians elsewhere. The bankruptcy has nothing to do with homeopathy; obviously such a large city hospital has been practicing mainstream medicine for decades—only the name has remained.

Could it possibly be time for some of the current skeptics to look into such historical details? As famous doctor and author Deepak Chopra puts it, these are "professional skeptics who are self-appointed vigilantes dedicated to the suppression of curiosity".[107]

Another group of professional skeptics is sitting around at Wikipedia. Wikipedia frequently headlines sections pertaining to controversial subjects with the words, "This section may lend undue weight to certain ideas, incidents, or controversies. Please help to create a more balanced presentation". Which, in my opinion, means it's juicy enough to dive right in.

This happened when I looked at the page of Nobel Prize in physiology or medicine 2008 winner Luc Montagnier, who—*somehow*—was exiled in China. What had happened? Of course, he had gone out on a limb—*way too far*! During the Lindau Nobel Laureate Meeting in Germany in 2010, he had spoken favorably about homeopathy in front of sixty other Nobel Prize winners and another 700 regular scientists![108] If he had thought he was big enough to say such frivolous things to these important people and go unpunished, he was clearly wrong. He was forced to pack up his things and go to China, where he's been successful as a professor at Shanghai Jiao Tong University. But Wikipedia coverage strictly ends with the "incident". So, what was it that he discovered that is so "out there"? It must have been along the lines

[107] Deepak Chopra, Huffpost, Dec 27, **2009**

[108] https://www.theaustralian.com.au/news/health-science/nobel-laureate-gives-homeopathy-a-boost/news-story/90fdf318d7ff067d6d23fbdb4fad955d

of "even if it were true, I wouldn't believe it".[109]

It turned out that Montagnier wasn't the only one who looked into the connection between water and electromagnetic waves, or some types of water memory. Jacques Benveniste had previously done it, publishing an article in the prestigious journal Nature in 1988, apparently endorsing homeopathy by claiming a special type of water memory exists. It's not clear what happened to the original article or if it was withdrawn, but let's just say that it was extremely unpleasant for everyone involved.

---

[109] Enserink, M. Newsmaker Interview: Luc Montagnier, French Nobelist Escapes "intellectual Terror" to Pursue Radical Ideas in China *Science* 24, December **2010**, *Vol 330(6012)*: 1732

mental
emotional
physical
DO YOU HAVE A DOCTOR'S NOTE? OTHERWISE YOU CAN'T BRING THIS ONTO THE PLANE...
HAVE YOU TRIED HOMEOPATHY? MY MOTHER THE QUEEN IS USING IT!
YES, I KNOW... THIS IS THE ONLY THING I CAN EAT...
Doctor's Note: patient is allergic to everything except for Rapunzel (rampion bellflower)
rapunzel
Epi-Pen
Allergy Meds

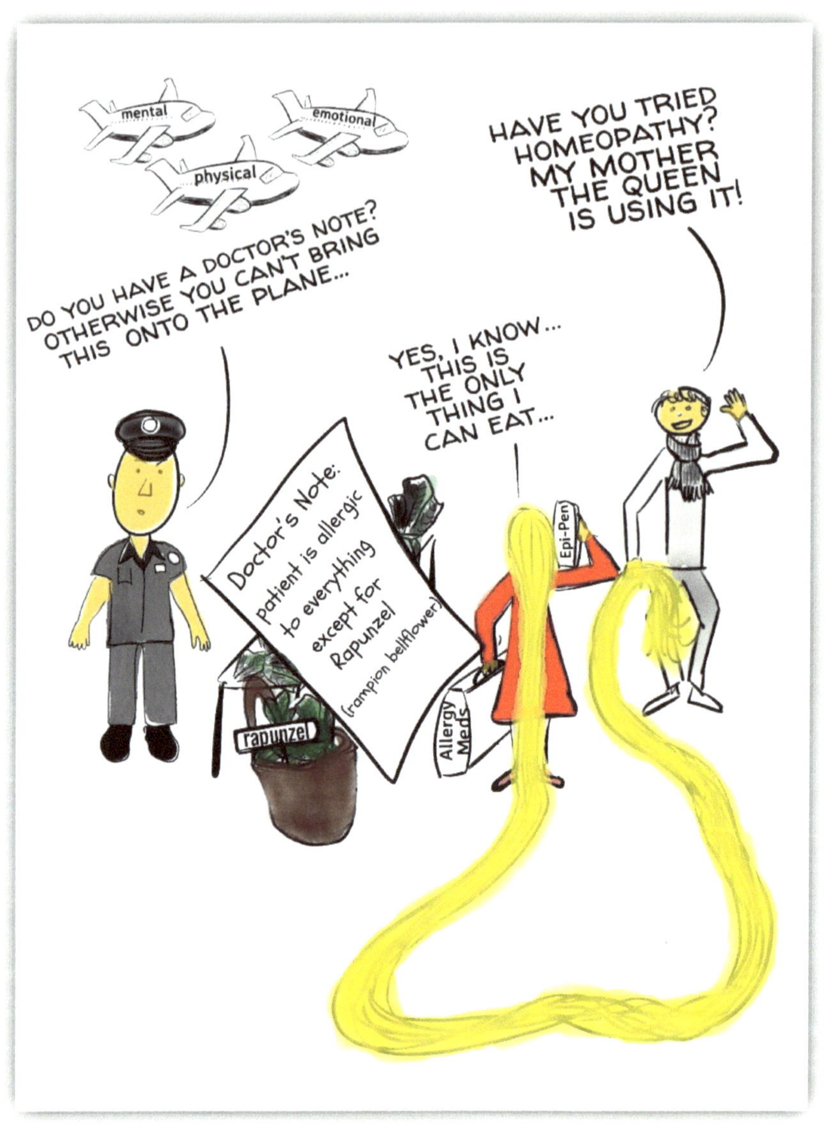

Homeopathic Fairy Tales:
Rapunzel

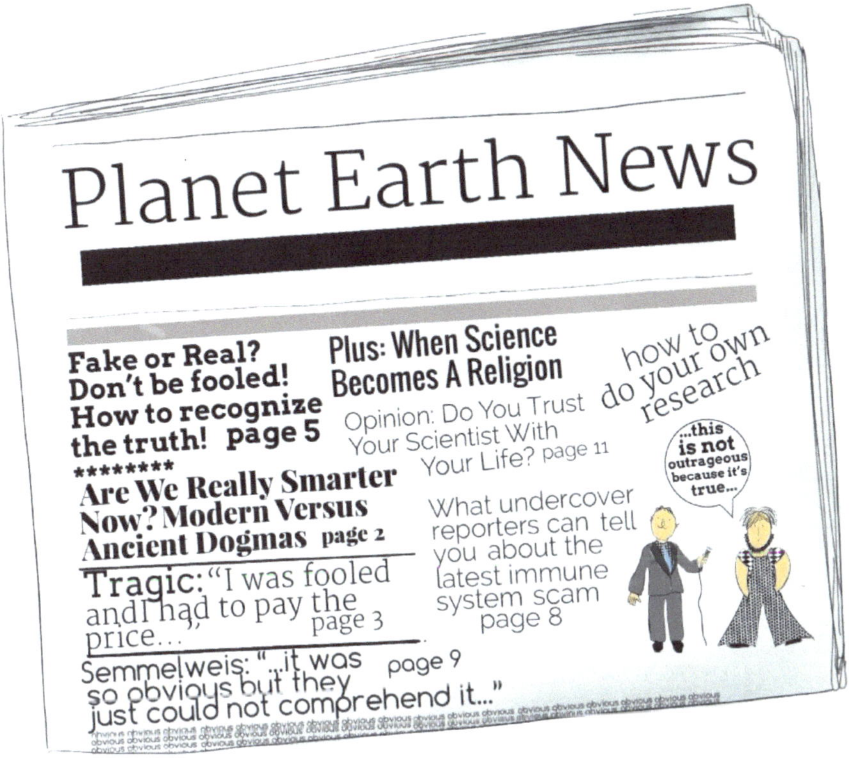

Planet Earth News

Fake or Real? Don't be fooled! How to recognize the truth! page 5

Plus: When Science Becomes A Religion

how to do your own research

Opinion: Do You Trust Your Scientist With Your Life? page 11

****

Are We Really Smarter Now? Modern Versus Ancient Dogmas page 2

...this is not outrageous because it's true...

Tragic: "I was fooled and I had to pay the price..." page 3

What undercover reporters can tell you about the latest immune system scam page 8

Semmelweis: "...it was so obvious but they just could not comprehend it..." page 9

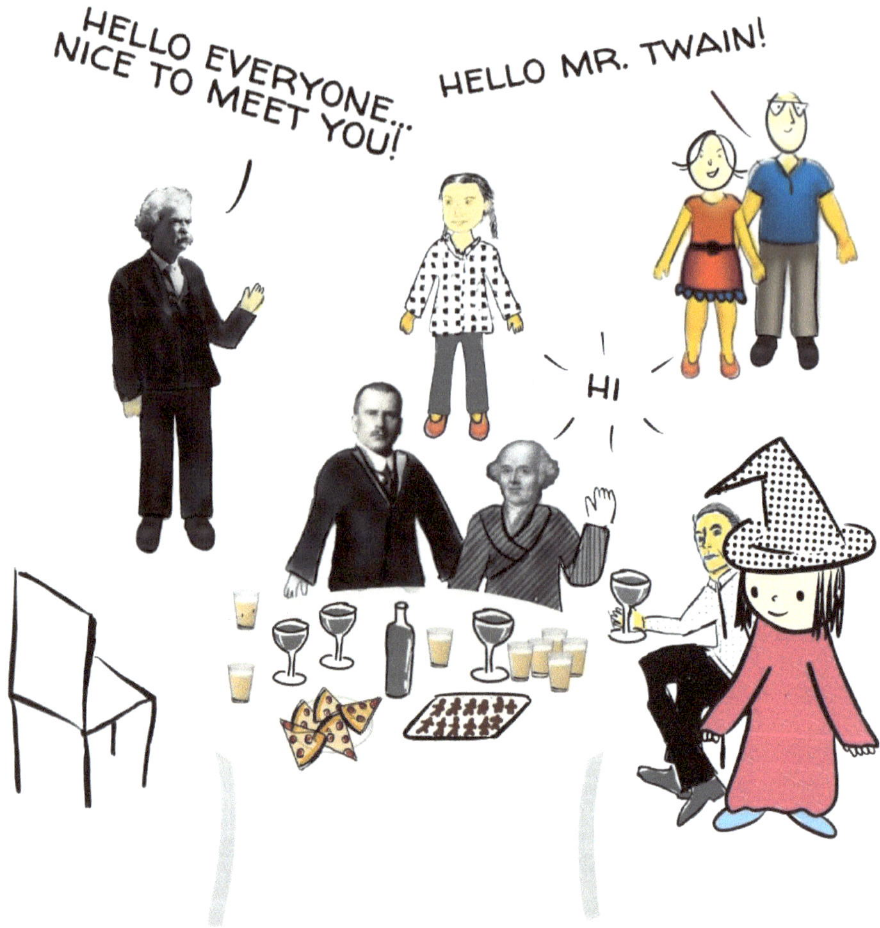
HELLO EVERYONE...
NICE TO MEET YOU!
HELLO MR. TWAIN!
HI

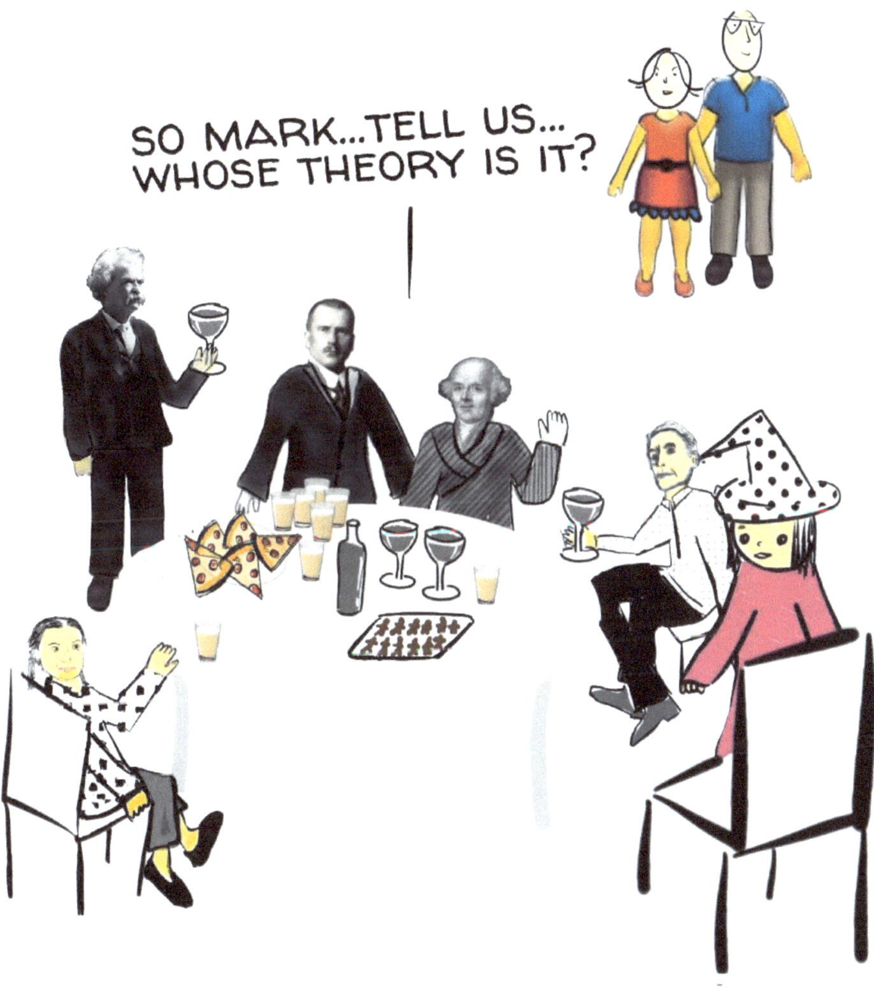
SO MARK...TELL US...
WHOSE THEORY IS IT?

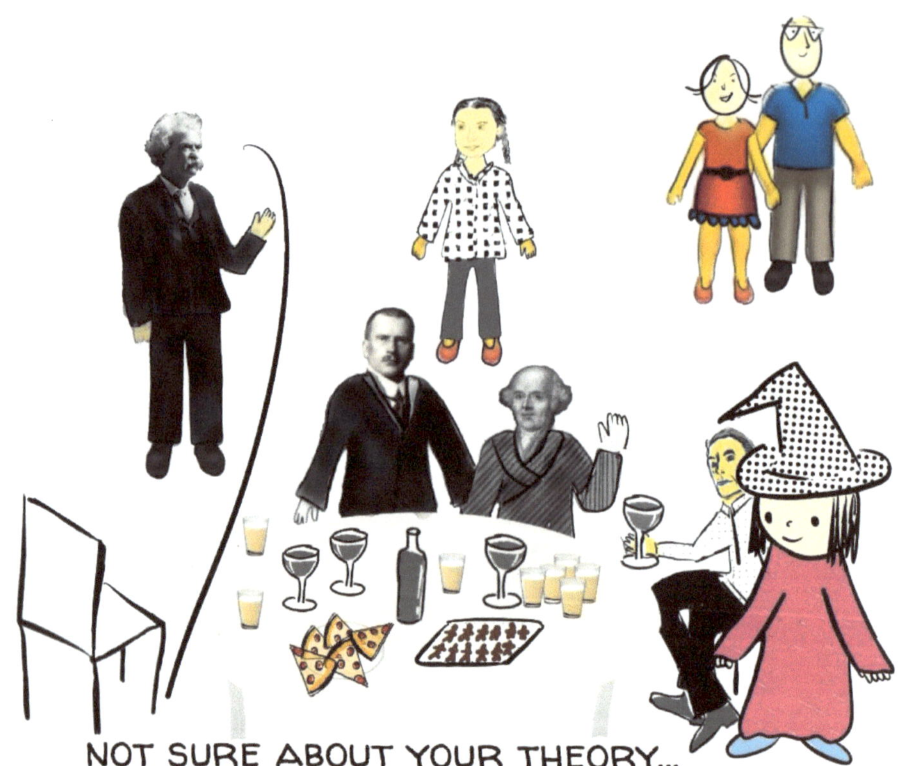

NOT SURE ABOUT YOUR THEORY...
BUT THE INTRODUCTION OF HOMEOPATHY
FORCED THE OLD SCHOOL DOCTOR TO STIR
AROUND AND LEARN SOMETHING OF A
RATIONAL NATURE ABOUT HIS BUSINESS...
YOU MAY HONESTLY FEEL GRATEFUL THAT
HOMEOPATHY SURVIVED THE ATTEMPTS
OF THE ALLOPATHS TO DESTROY IT...

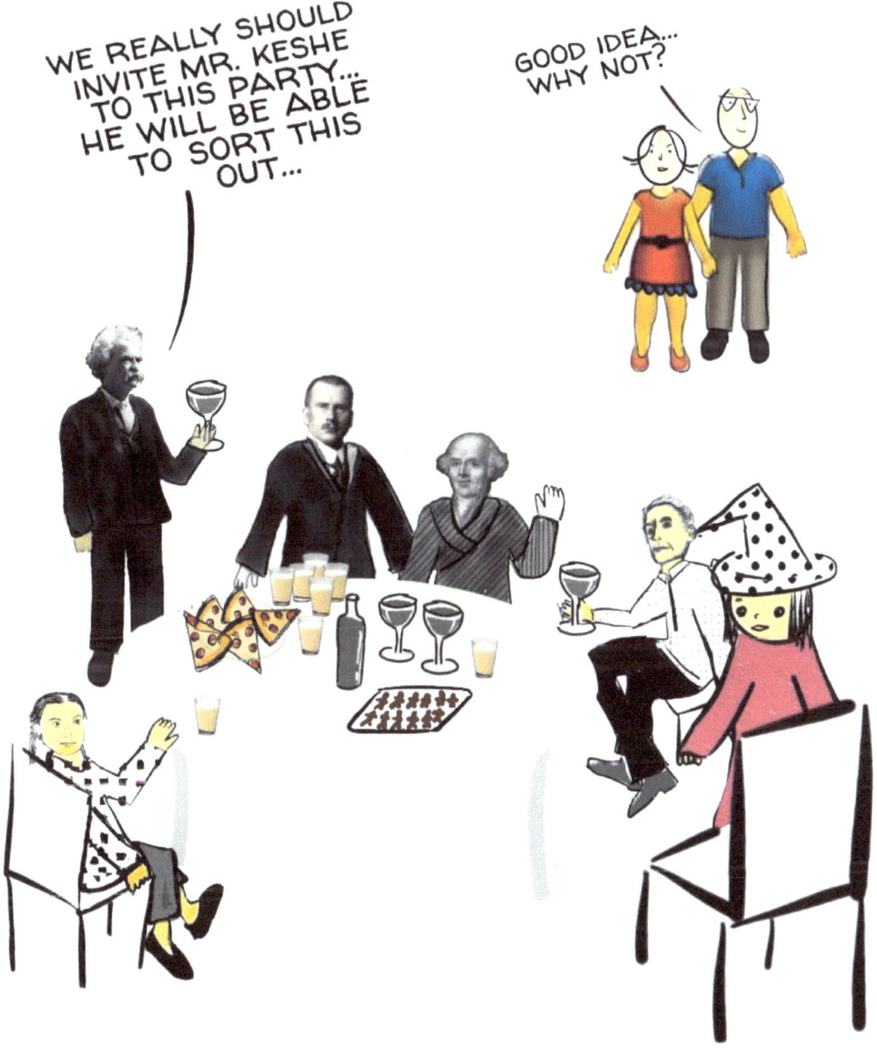
WE REALLY SHOULD INVITE MR. KESHE TO THIS PARTY... HE WILL BE ABLE TO SORT THIS OUT...
GOOD IDEA... WHY NOT?

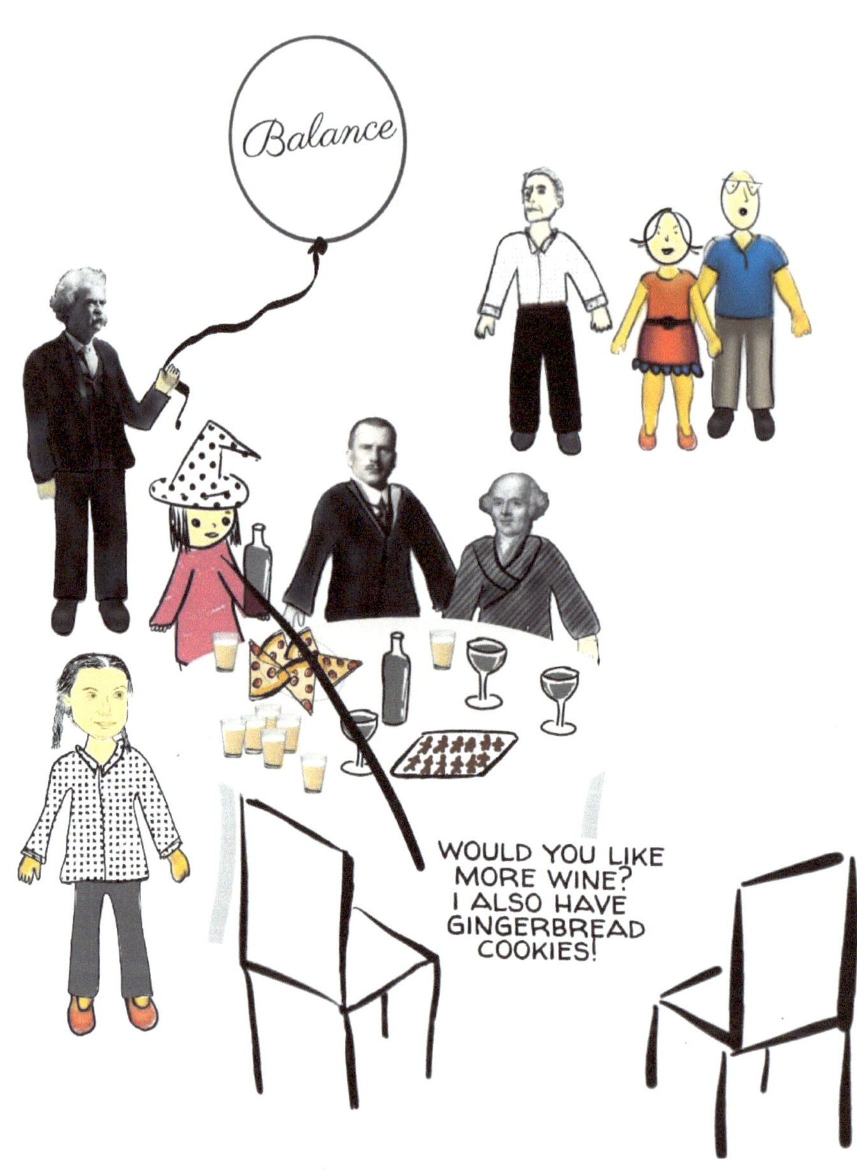
Balance
WOULD YOU LIKE
MORE WINE?
I ALSO HAVE
GINGERBREAD
COOKIES!

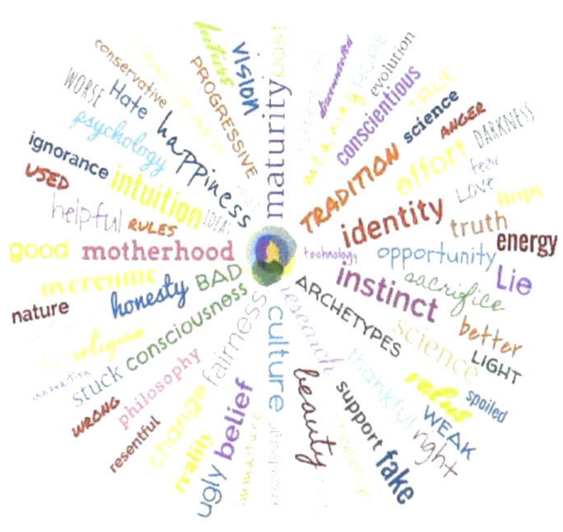
maturity
vision
PROGRESSIVE
conservative
WORSE
Hate
happiness
psychology
ignorance
USED
intuition
helpful
RULES
good
motherhood
nature
honesty
BAD
consciousness
stuck
philosophy
WRONG
resentful
change
fairness
culture
belief
ugly
research
beauty
support
fake
WEAK
right
spoiled
LIGHT
better
science
ARCHETYPES
instinct
sacrifice
Lie
opportunity
technology
identity
truth
energy
TRADITION
effort
science
ANGER
DARKNESS
LOVE
conscientious
evolution
HOPE
TRUE

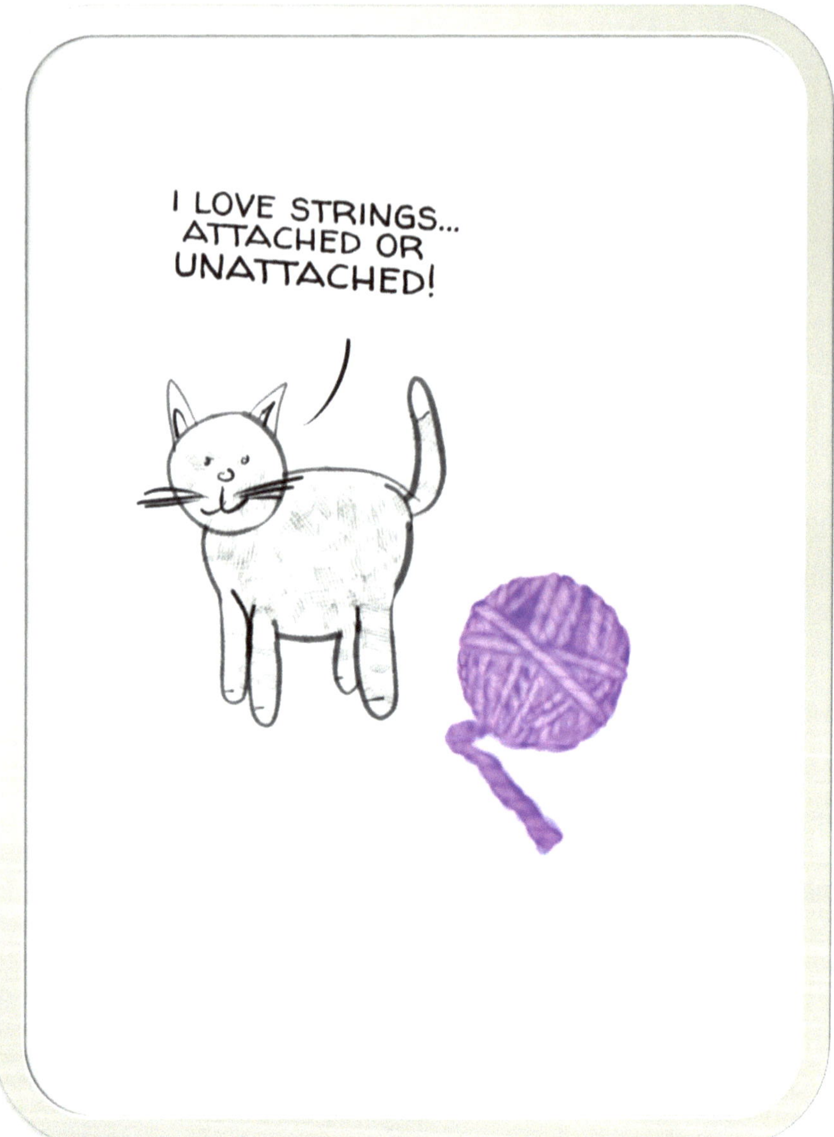
I LOVE STRINGS...
ATTACHED OR
UNATTACHED!

Forget String Theory

By Misna Burelli

Now, several years into this quest, if there was a pattern through it all, it was this: water was at least partially responsible for the effects of homeopathy. Water—an unusual molecule, with its density anomaly preventing the oceans from freezing up, allowing aquatic life to thrive, even in the deepest depths. On top of that, it was a dipole—a polar molecule, perfectly positioned to act as life's primary solvent everywhere, from oceans to blood vessels. At the cellular level, the newly discovered 4th phase helped explain the cell membrane potential effect. But even with all these unusual characteristics, nothing I could find, up to this point, could explain homeopathic effects in water solutions.

Imagine my surprise then, when, after all this tedious and confusing research, I came across a simple article on the internet, titled: *The Unknown Truth about Homeopathy* by Mehran Keshe.[110] In the fifteen page paper, he explains that homeopathy is actually a form of magnetism. All matter can be categorized into ferromagnetic, paramagnetic or diamagnetic materials and is therefore susceptible to being magnetized by a surrounding field.

Most of us are familiar with common ferromagnetic materials, such as refrigerator magnets, but these weaker forms of magnetism—paramagnetism and diamagnetism—follow similar rules.

So, how would magnetism impact our bodies, and how would a remedy become magnetized? Pretty simple actually: any magnetic material can be magnetized further by impact. Hitting a nail with a hammer perpendicular to Earth's magnetic field will eventually create a small magnet. You can try to do this yourself—it's not difficult![111]

Shaking a liquid filled container perpendicular to Earth's magnetic field will also create a magnet, as long as the solution contains entities that can be magnetized. And yes, the magnetic forces that we are

110 Keshefoundation.org

111 https://www.wikihow.com/Magnetize-Metal and https://www.wikihow.com/Magnetize-Steel

talking about here are *tiny*. In the case of a solution, the magnetization will bring out an alignment that only gets *stronger* through subsequent *dilution* and additional *shaking*—homeopathic succussion. And after the water solution has been magnetized, the original solute molecule is not even needed anymore—exactly as expected in homeopathy! This is precisely how homeopathic remedies are made: by shaking or—as instructed in the original texts by Hahnemann—by hitting a leather-bound book with a sturdy glass vessel, containing the remedy solution. It's clearly similar to striking a nail with a hammer, although done more gently by hitting a book. And because the human body has its own magnetic field, it would obviously react to a magnetic solution with its own realignment, in a way that might be beneficial.

Even though the magnetic fields that are produced through this process are very small, it seems the human body is sensitive enough to pick up these tiny fields and to work with them. Some people are more sensitive than others. This is common knowledge in homeopathy, and the reason why homeopathic potencies—*magnetic strengths*—of remedies are adjusted to match an ailment or the particular health condition of a client.

If you have ever taken a homeopathic remedy, you know that it works *immediately*—within seconds. As soon as your tongue touches the remedy, the headache might be gone! It follows that homeopathy must be based on a mechanism that can be felt instantly, without digestion or metabolic activation—just like the influence of a magnetic field!

This sounds pretty straightforward, and the fact that humans have their own magnetic fields should not come as a surprise. After all, living within Earth's magnetic field constantly magnetizes the human body. The magnetic misalignments occurring as a result of disease, injuries, and interference by other magnetic fields might be the true culprits preventing perfect health. Using a magnetic solution to realign mistuned parts is exactly what we should be doing!

But what about the little white pills? They are dry! Yes, they are dry, but only after having been soaked in the magnetized remedy solution—*then they are dried*. They are just a carrier material for magnetism. This also explains how it has been possible for homeopaths to extend their old remedies simply by adding new clean sugar pills to the old bottle! After mixing them all and shaking them up a few times, the new remedy is as good as the old one! This has been a dirty little secret that people liked to avoid—no one could explain it, but somehow everyone always knew that it worked! It was kept a secret because it was clear that it would undermine the credibility of homeopathy even more. Now it makes perfect sense! It is identical in its principle to magnetizing a new nail with a previously magnetized nail—a commonly known phenomenon.

Or how about the information that people who receive a heart transplant often take on parts of the personality of the organ donor? Even though this could involve more complicated details than just a magnetic field, the idea that the field of the donor would rub off on the receiver seems like a good starting hypothesis to me.

And finally, the last perfectly fitting piece of the puzzle is of course—*you guessed it*—polarity. Polarity, observable in homeopathic remedies, has its matching counterpart in the plus and minus poles of magnetic fields: there is attraction and repulsion, pulling and pushing. Magnetic fields are a form of polarity, they are centered on that basic science concept.

Sounds too easy to be true? I had to admit, I wanted to be skeptical, even though the magnetic field explanation sounded plausible and its simplicity was elegant. And just to clarify: we should always be skeptical, especially when proposing new ideas or hypotheses, but at the same time, we should be open minded enough to allow ourselves to look for new solutions—even if they are a bit "out there". We should not discard any kind of science that we simply don't *yet* understand, can't make a profit off of, or just dislike, in favor of keeping the status quo.

Besides, this explanation is well within scientific principles, and the author is not even a homeopath, but rather a nuclear physicist—a clear bonus! Obviously, he had read through all of Samuel Hahnemann's original publications from two hundred years ago, but he interpreted them with a scientist's eye.

I contacted the publishing organization and inquired about their copyright status, patents etc. Here is how they responded: *"Follow your heart!"*

So, I have been following my heart, trying to bring this information out into the open where it is urgently needed. I hope you will follow your heart as well, spreading this knowledge and making a difference in the world—no strings attached!

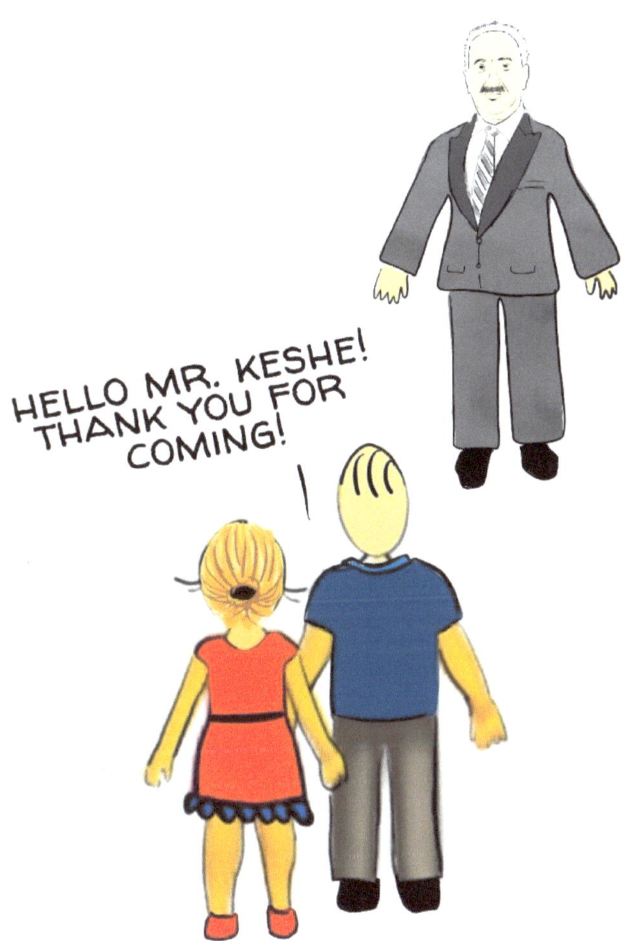
HELLO MR. KESHE!
THANK YOU FOR
COMING!

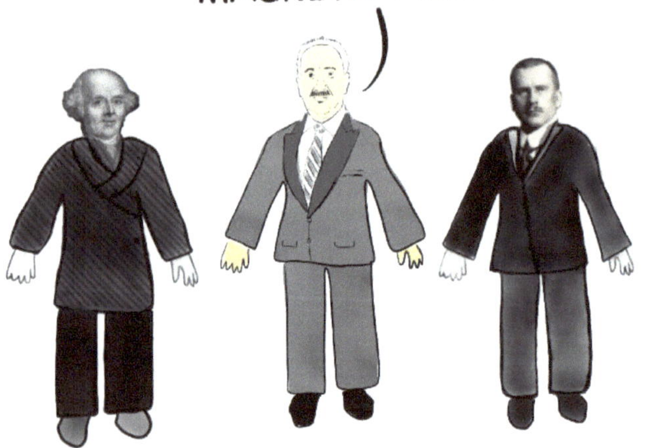
ABOUT YOUR THEORIES...
YOU ARE BOTH RIGHT...
THERE IS NO NEED TO ARGUE
BECAUSE RATHER THAN ARGUING,
WE SHOULD FOCUS ON THE FUTURE...
THERE IS SO MUCH TO EXPLORE,
NOW THAT WE KNOW ABOUT
THE POWER OF THE
MAGNETIC FIELDS!

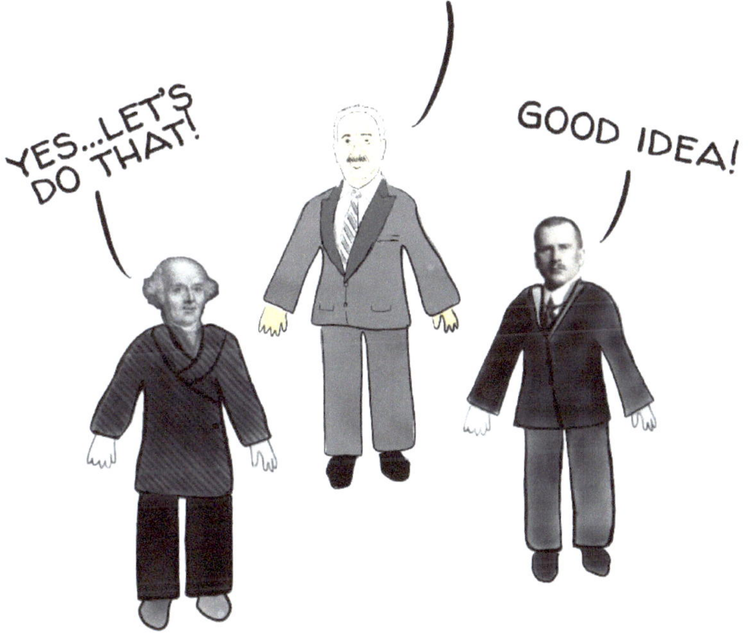
LET'S TAKE A WALK...
AND LET'S TALK...
YES...LET'S DO THAT!
GOOD IDEA!

...THERE IS WITHIN AN IRON BAR... A SLUMBERING TRACE OF MAGNETIC FORCE...WHEN IT HAS BEEN LEFT STANDING UPRIGHT IMMEDIATELY AFTER BEING FORGED, ITS LOWER END REPELS THE NORTH POLE OF A MAGNETIC NEEDLE AND ATTRACTS THE SOUTH POLE

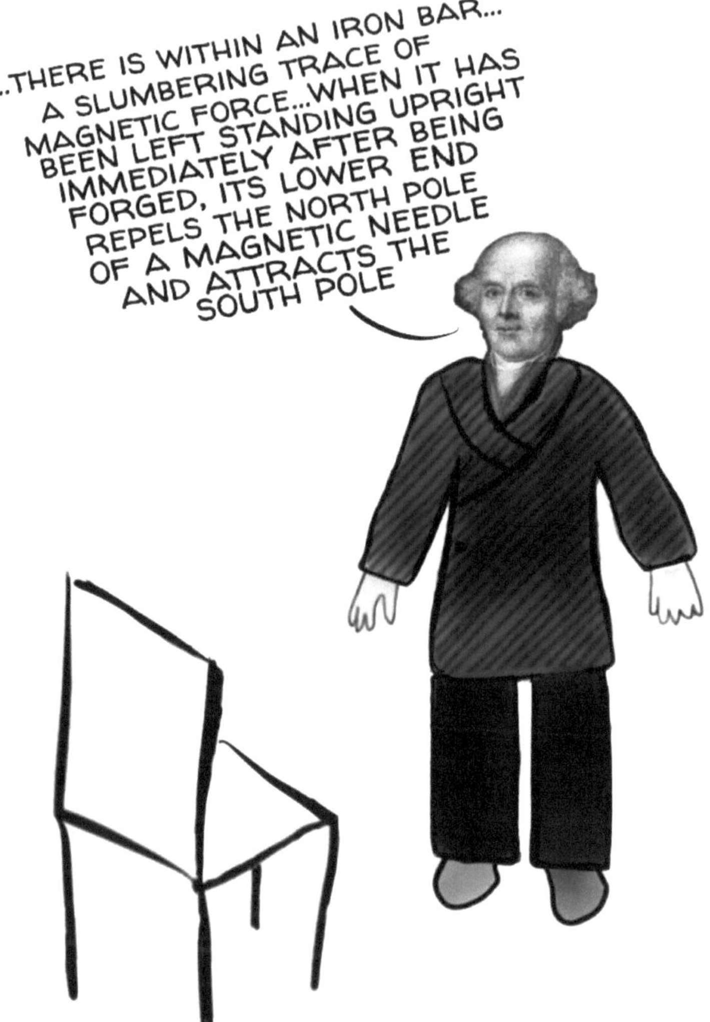

From Organon Of Medicine [112]

[112] Hahnemann, S. *Organon of Medicine,* Koethen, Germany, **1810**, *Aph. 269*

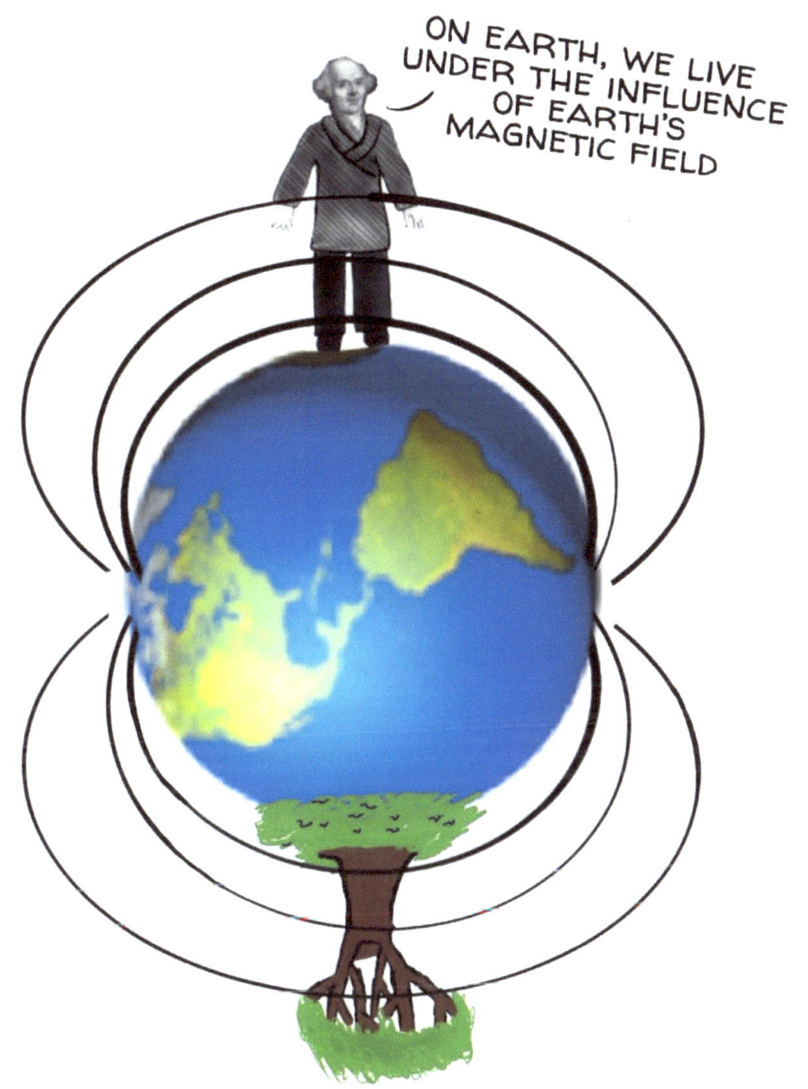
ON EARTH, WE LIVE UNDER THE INFLUENCE OF EARTH'S MAGNETIC FIELD

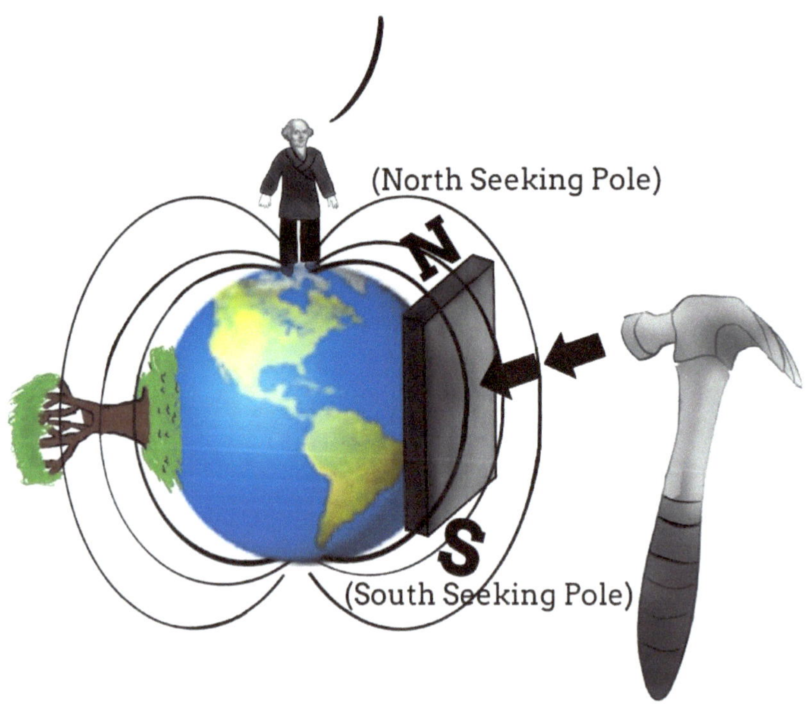
HITTING AN IRON PIECE REPEATEDLY WITH A HAMMER, WHILE UNDER THE INFLUENCE OF A MAGNETIC FIELD, WILL MAKE IT MAGNETIC BECAUSE THE VIBRATION CAUSES THE MANY SMALL MAGNETIC DOMAINS TO REARRANGE THEMSELVES
(North Seeking Pole)
N
S
(South Seeking Pole)

A SOLUTION IS
MAGNETIZED BY HITTING A
GLASS VESSEL AGAINST
A "LEATHER BOUND BOOK"

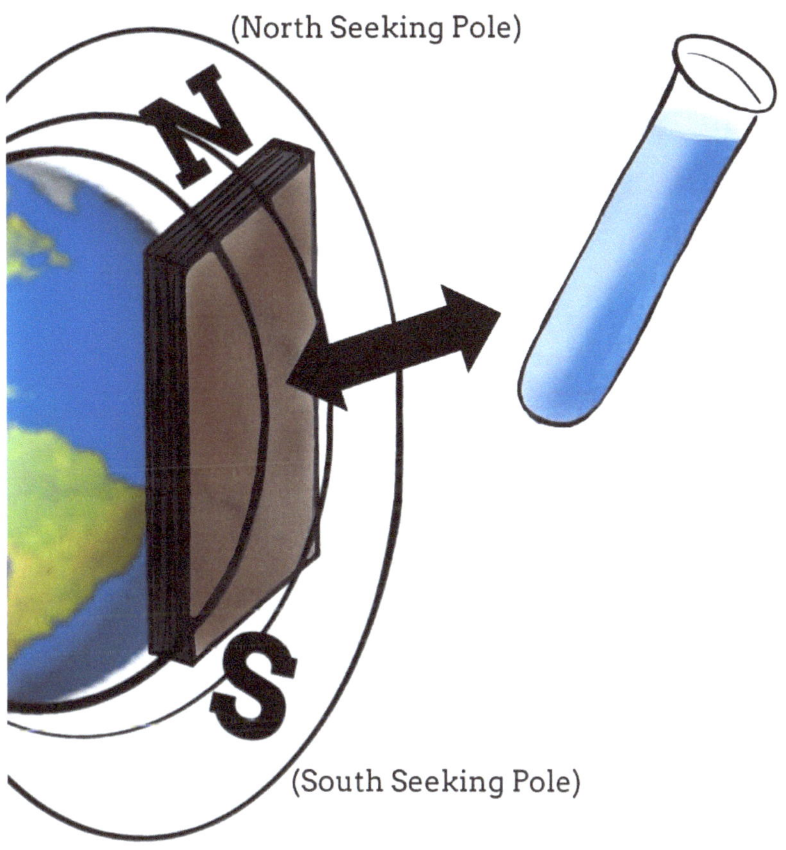

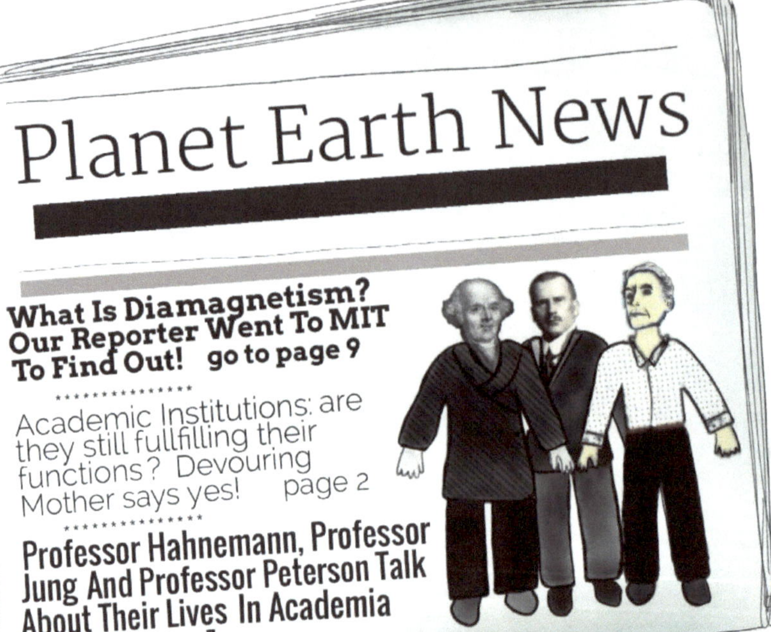
Planet Earth News
What Is Diamagnetism? Our Reporter Went To MIT To Find Out! go to page 9
Academic Institutions: are they still fullfilling their functions? Devouring Mother says yes! page 2
Professor Hahnemann, Professor Jung And Professor Peterson Talk About Their Lives In Academia
full report on page 7

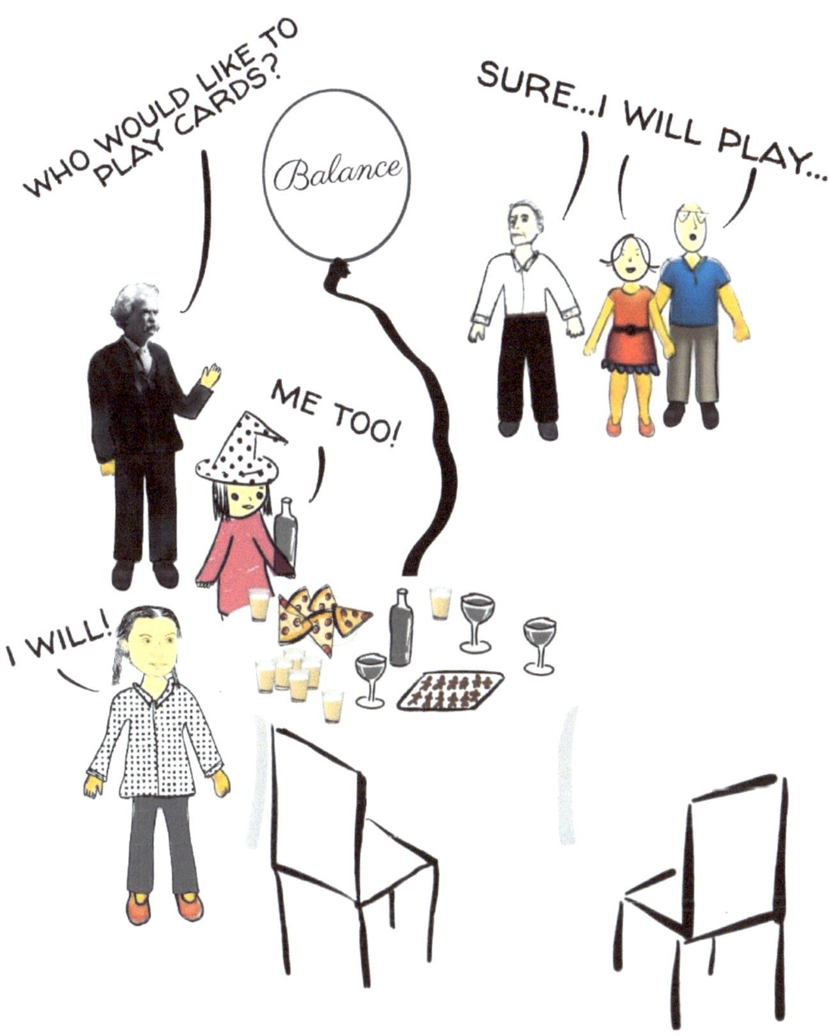
WHO WOULD LIKE TO PLAY CARDS?
Balance
SURE...I WILL PLAY...
ME TOO!
I WILL!

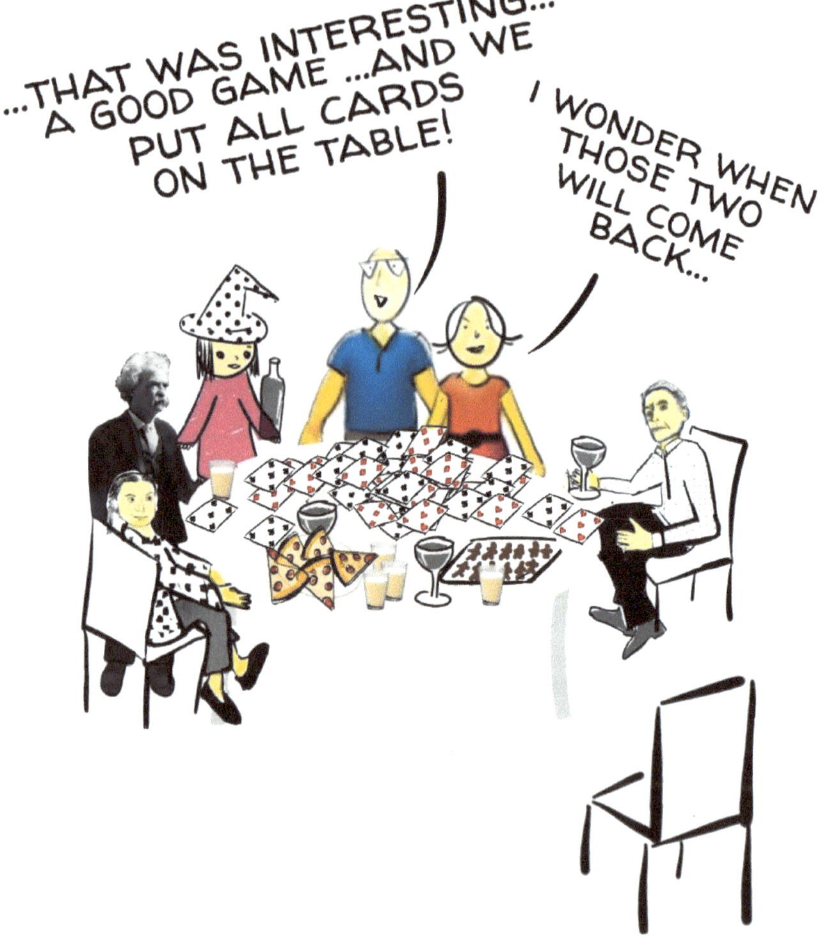
...THAT WAS INTERESTING...
A GOOD GAME ...AND WE
PUT ALL CARDS
ON THE TABLE!
I WONDER WHEN
THOSE TWO
WILL COME
BACK...

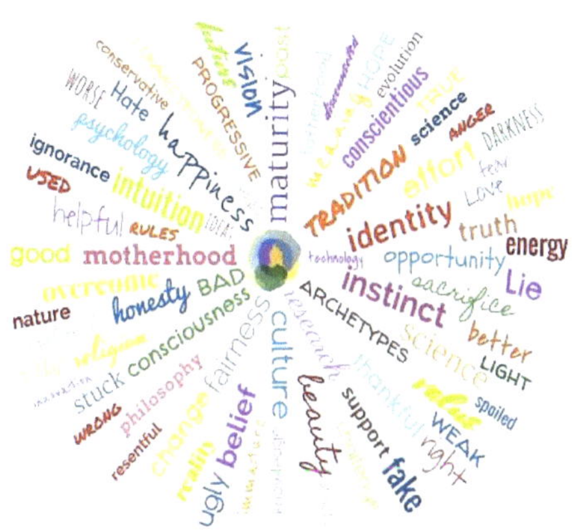
conservative
WORSE
Hate
psychology
ignorance
USED
helpful
RULES
intuition
happiness
PROGRESSIVE
VISION
maturity
evolution
HOPE
conscientious
science
ANGER
DARKNESS
TRADITION
effort
Love
hope
identity
truth
energy
technology
opportunity
Lie
good
motherhood
nature
honesty
BAD
consciousness
instinct
sacrifice
ARCHETYPES
science
better
LIGHT
stuck
philosophy
fairness
culture
beauty
thankful
values
spoiled
WRONG
resentful
change
belief
support
WEAK
right
fake
ugly

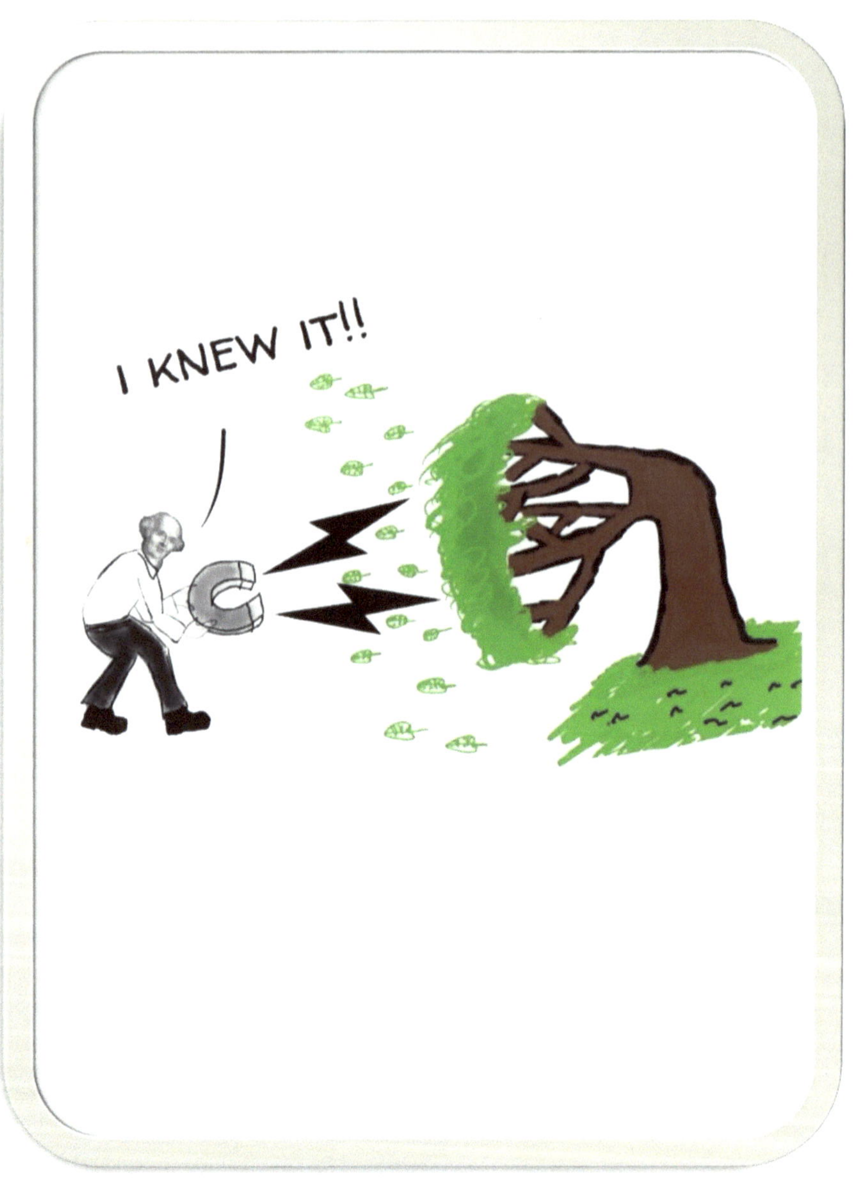
I KNEW IT!!

A New Paradigm

By Lena Kratz

So where do we go from here? Straight to more research! For a long time, I have waited for the mystery of homeopathy to be solved. I am convinced it will bring a revolution of major technological advancements in not only medicine, but also other disciplines—*a paradigm shift.* Similarly to how the internet and digital revolution shaped a whole new era of communication and commerce, the idea of applying magnetic fields as new healing tools must be a springboard for further exploration. Even though it seems intuitively correct to assume that the human body would automatically be imprinted with magnetic fields, we are still far away from understanding even the basics. Which magnetic fields might be beneficial? How strong should a field be? How do magnetic fields interact with each other, contributing to health or disease?

Going back to some of the archetype examples from earlier chapters, we could ask if miasms—the "old imprints", which can be observed in large parts of the population—are in fact previously magnetically mistuned parts of the human body. As magnetic fields they could easily be carried on for generations, invariably transferring from mother and father to their offspring.

And we could also ask if acute diseases, such as measles, might carry magnetic fields with them, "infecting" certain parts of the population—the ones with no previous exposure to the disease. It might not be such a farfetched idea to speculate that "catching" acute diseases could help with magnetically retuning the body. In fact, it would fit right in with previously mentioned research, suggesting measles and other acute illnesses are protective against cancer and other disease states.

Let's see what happens when we apply the hypothesis of "invisible" magnetic fields as the origin of acute "similar" diseases: giving a matching homeopathic magnetic field remedy during the acute phase of the disease can be of great assistance. As stated earlier, some acute diseases with very well-known remedy pictures constantly seem to circle the earth, reappearing seasonally. This is true for the combinations of measles and *pulsatilla* or influenza and *rhus tox*, and also others. Assuming that homeopathy is mainly a magnetic field, it seems not too far-fetched to speculate that one field would influence the other, leading to a dramatic improvement in symptoms or speeding up recovery. Assimilating those fields might result in the aforementioned deep retuning of the human body, a process that would be protective on a physical, emotional, and mental level, helping to clear out old magnetic imbalances.

Admittedly, there are not a lot of peer reviewed data supporting the magnetic field theory of homeopathy—*yet*. But I fully expect any future evidence to be overwhelming. Why am I so confident? It is because all the loose ends have been tied up—there are no holes or mismatched parts—everything fits together exactly how it should. Like a glove on a hand. The theory simply resonates on a level never seen before. It beautifully explains away many of the original problems associated with homeopathy, but most importantly, it deals with the *conundrum* of *"not containing anything"*.

Last but not least, it also allows homeopaths to put the ball back in the court of the people who constantly claim to protect consumers from the scam that is homeopathy, entirely without ever researching it. But since it is difficult to defend a product without being able to present a scientific mechanism—an accepted theory—those people always look like very legitimate fighters for the common good.

Homeopathy distributors have had to continually battle lawsuits over the sale of their frequently successful products, even though they have been regulated by the FDA and follow their labeling requirements. Rather than leaving the choice up to the consumer, certain groups would like to make decisions for everyone—or is it just a deep seated *fear of change*?[113]

But maybe it's time for a challenge. Now, with a hypothetical mechanism behind homeopathy, perhaps we should consider what

---

113 Johnson, S. *Who Moved My Cheese? An Amazing Way to Deal With Change In Your Work and In Your Life* Random House, London, **1998**

happens when some people *miss out* on the lifesaving treatment that could be homeopathy. At least there should be a choice that comes with *informed consent*—the basis of all ethical medicine. And maybe all this is happening at a critical time. With antibiotic resistance ever increasing, we will soon be desperate for new treatment options that are independent of those failing drugs.

But back to magnetic field therapy. There have been other magnetic stimulation treatments available for years,[114] with Amazon carrying a whole range of "pain relief" magnets, magnetic wraps, and magnetic acupuncture point spot patches. Maybe they are on to something?

So, what is the connection between magnetic fields, human disease, and archetypes, such as the Devouring Mother? Is it possible to get contaminated with one magnetic field and decontaminated with another? The question of how it is all interrelated begs to be answered! We should be open to addressing these matters while creating a *truly diverse* field of scientific inquiry, which is not limited by preconceived notions of politically correct research. As a culture and scientific community, we need to get away from the paradigm of looking only for things that we can see with our eyes.

We should create a positive, welcoming environment—ideas need room to flow freely! Magnetic field research must become a starting point—*a platform*—to kick off more investigations, not only into archetypes but also polarity, voltages, and energy.

Many more questions will need to be asked and answered. There seems to be a lot of potential going beyond healthcare! Putting magnetic field research at the center of new innovations in transportation and energy research could open up whole new areas of development. We might be on the cusp of great discoveries! Really, this is *just the beginning*!

---

[114]Thinkingmomsrevolution.com/transcranial-magnetic-stimulation-son-autism-happened/

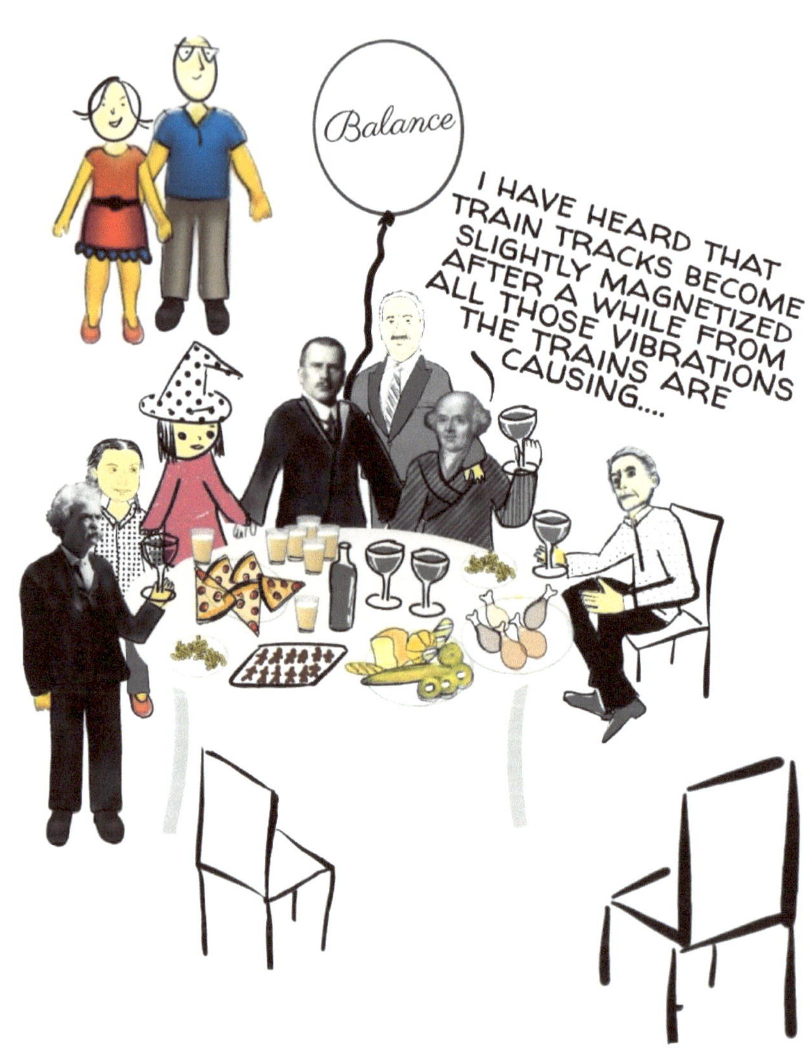
Balance
I HAVE HEARD THAT TRAIN TRACKS BECOME SLIGHTLY MAGNETIZED AFTER A WHILE FROM ALL THOSE VIBRATIONS THE TRAINS ARE CAUSING....

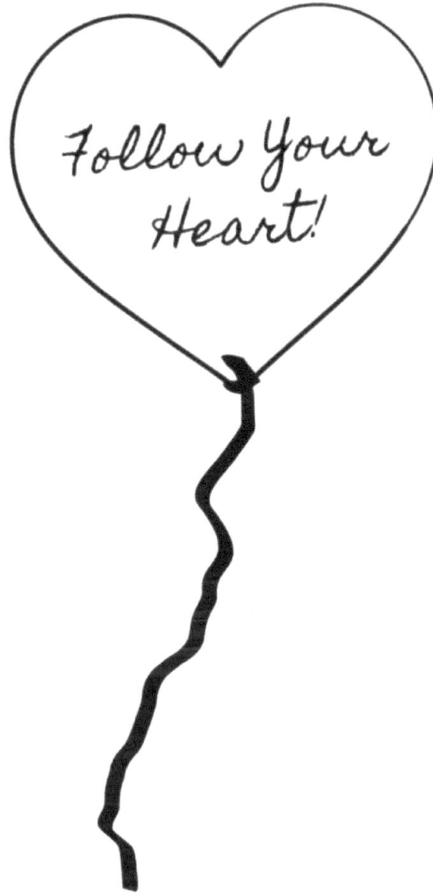
Follow Your
Heart!

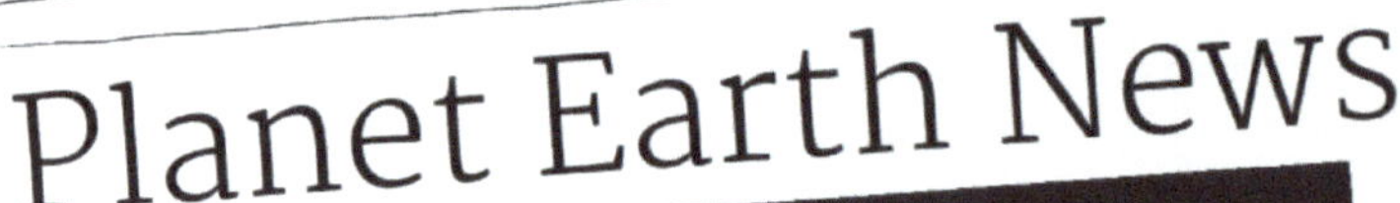

Planet Earth News

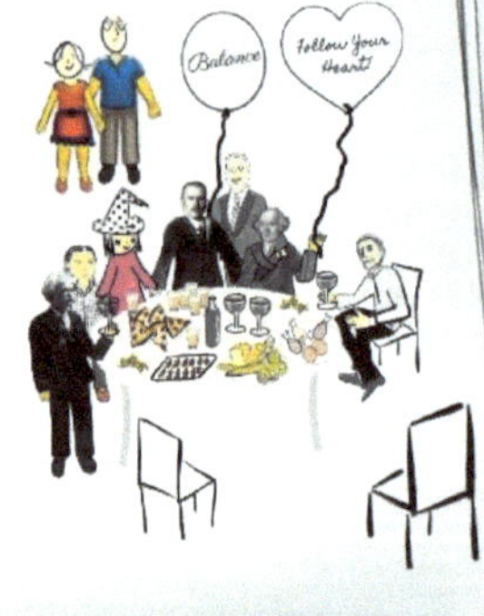

Group Picture At Mother Nature's: A Happy Ending!

****

Amazing: How One Party Can Change The World! page 3

Party Planning Secrets from Lena and Misna page 2

****

Mother Nature: Thank You For Coming, Future Looks Bright! page 11

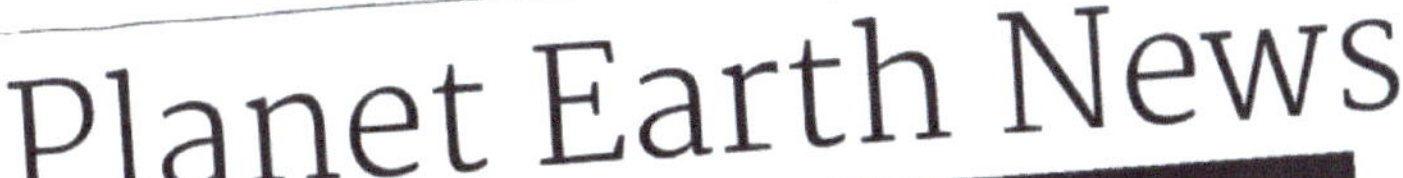

Planet Earth News

Paradigm Shift?
Mother Nature Says Yes!

Paradigm shift makes Mother Nature very happy.
See page 5 for excting new details!

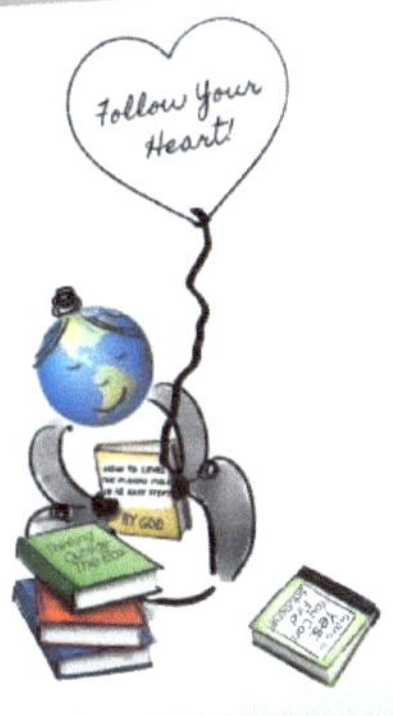

Party a great success!

New hope for humanity revealed.
Read all about it on page 6
New hope for humanity revealed. New hope for humanity revealed
New hope for humanity revealed. New hope for humanity revealed

New Inventions Forthcoming

New hope for humanity revealed. New hope for humanity revealed
New hope for humanity revealed. New hope for humanity revealed
New hope for humanity revealed Success stories take over the world!

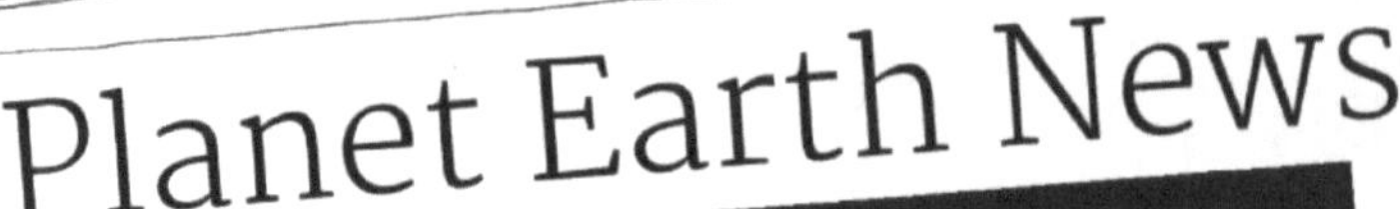
Planet Earth News
Best Friends: Hahnemann and Jung open up about how they found each other
On working together in the future: "will be fun...we know our theory is solid!"
exclusive details on page 11
New Hope For The Future: "All Credit Should Go To Mr. Keshe!"
Mother Nature: "game changer... extremely happy with outcome..."

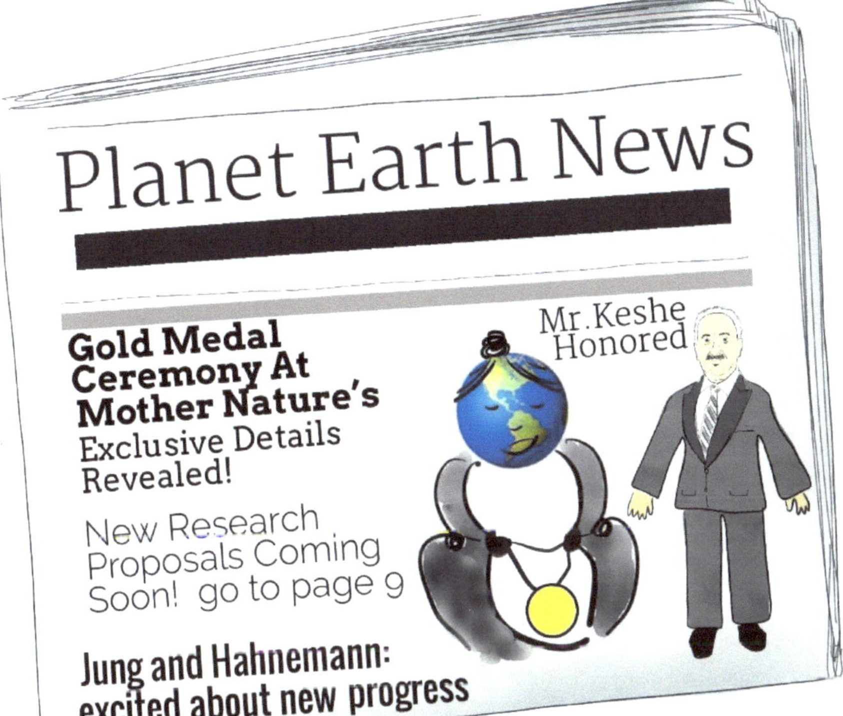
Planet Earth News
Gold Medal Ceremony At Mother Nature's
Exclusive Details Revealed!
New Research Proposals Coming Soon! go to page 9
Jung and Hahnemann: excited about new progress
Mr.Keshe Honored

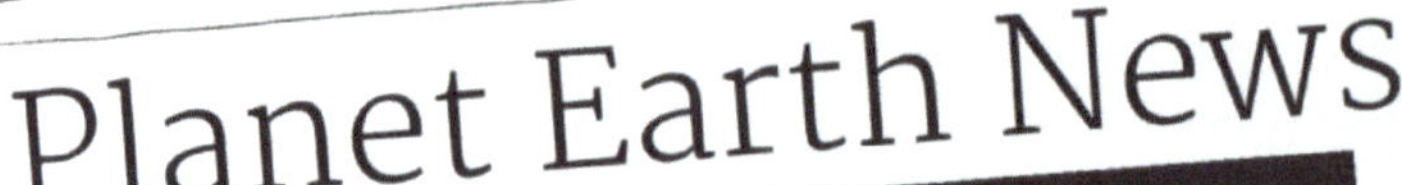

Planet Earth News

Good News: Magnetic Field Tech Boom Will Solve World's Problems! Go To Page 10 For A Full Report

****

Universities Announce Interest In Magnetic Field Research

****

Exciting New Developments: A Reason For Humanity To Come Together? page 5

****

Department Head: No Time for Identity Politics - Busy Planning For The Future page 9

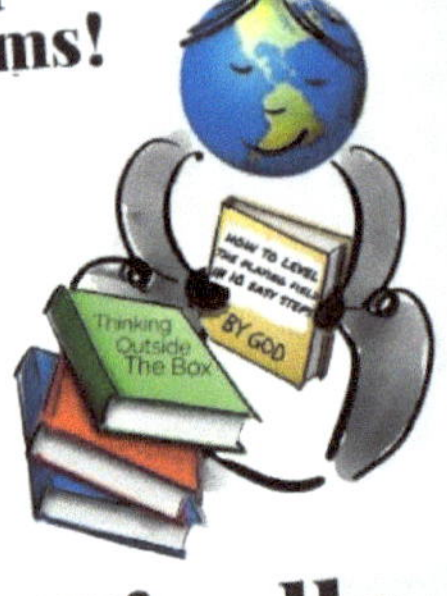

"Finally..."

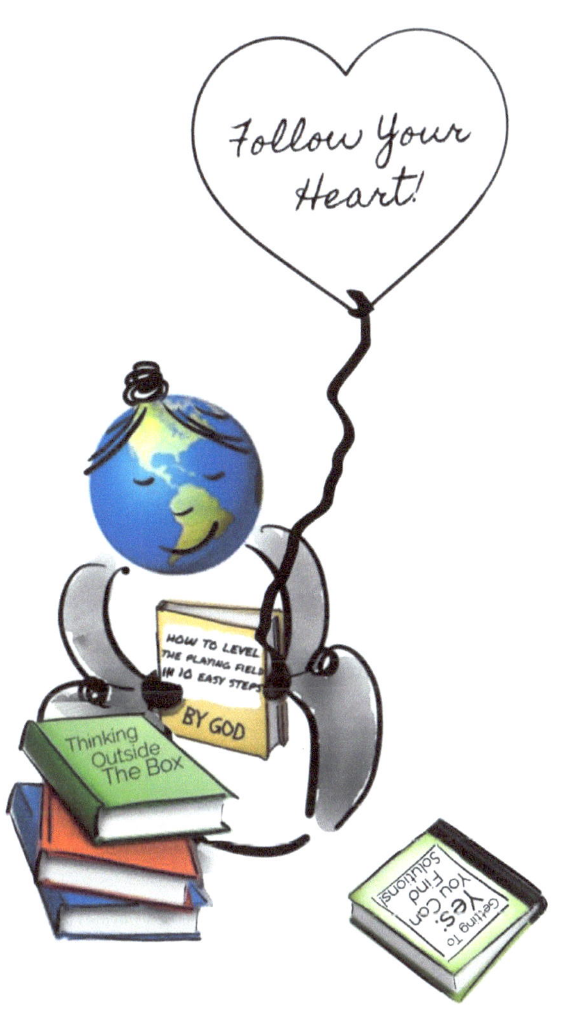
Follow Your Heart!
HOW TO LEVEL THE PLAYING FIELD IN 10 EASY STEPS
BY GOD
Thinking Outside The Box
Getting To Yes: You Can Find Solutions!

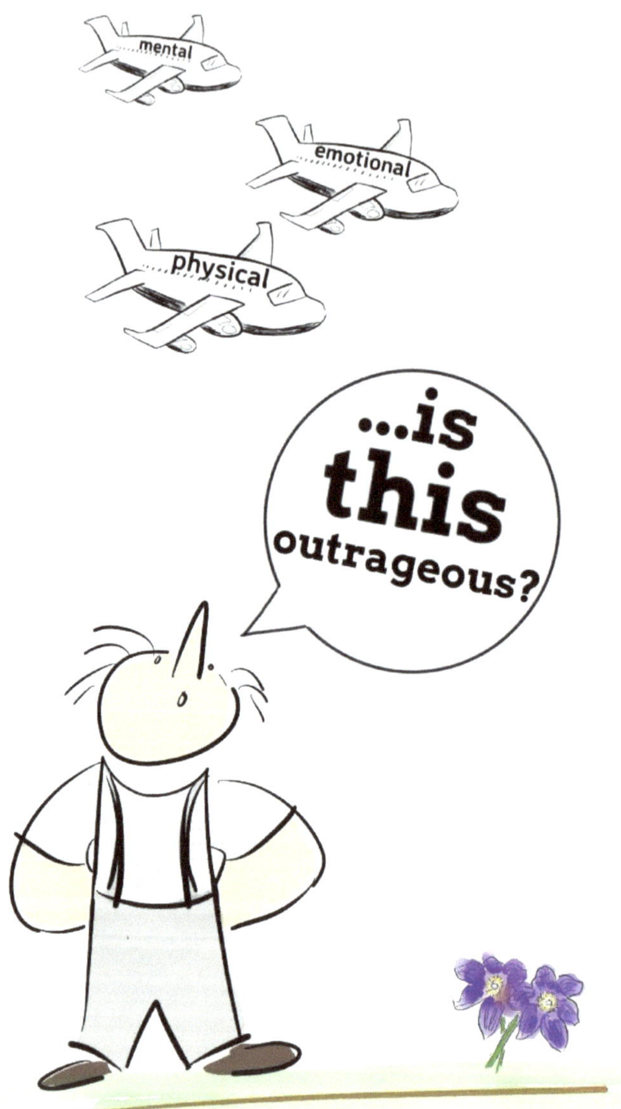
mental
emotional
physical
...is
this
outrageous?

Polarized

a Tragicomedy
in XVIII Parts

The End

WHAT A GOOD SHOW!
YES...I REALLY LIKED IT! GOOD ENDING TOO!

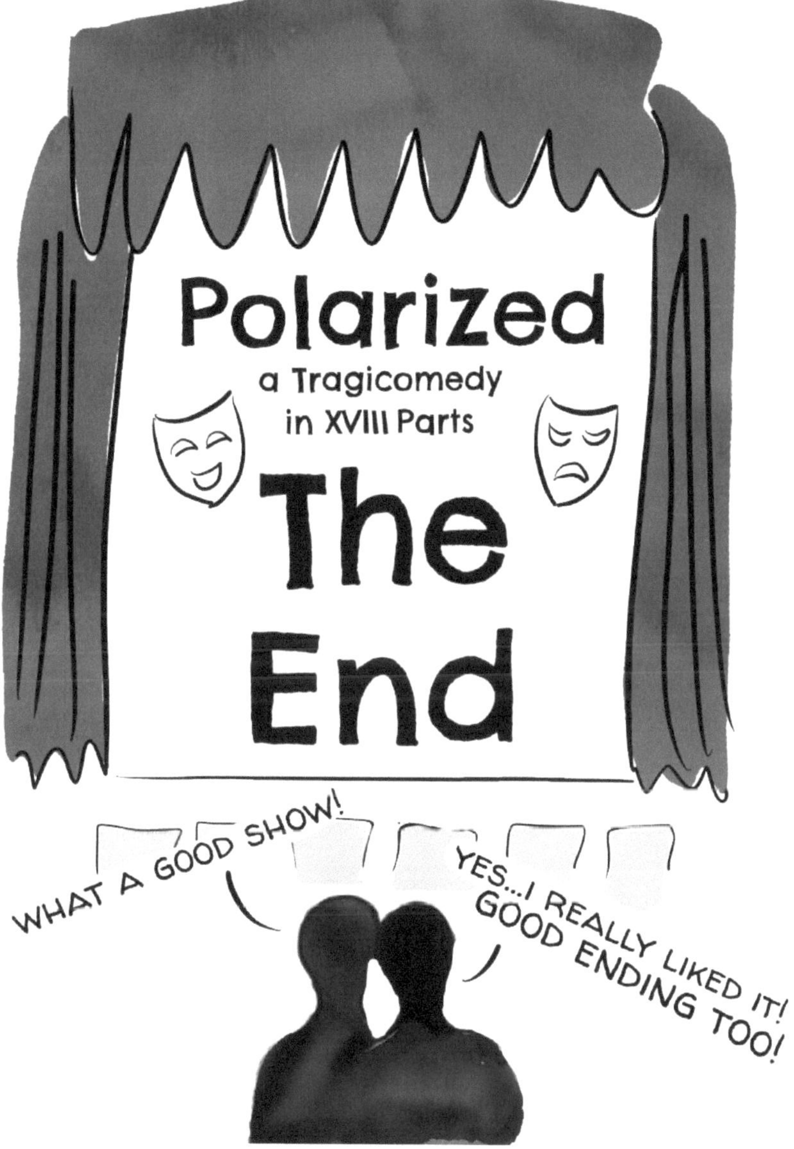

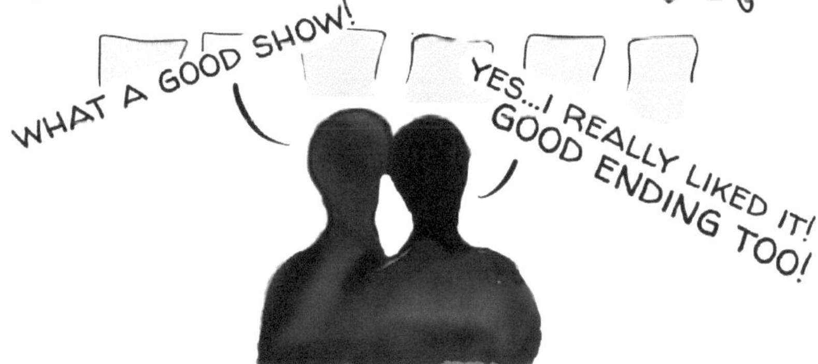

Index

www.ingramcontent.com/pod-product-compliance
Lightning Source LLC
LaVergne TN
LVHW072029110826
845147LV00001BA/2